Carville

Carville

REMEMBERING
LEPROSY IN
AMERICA

MARCIA GAUDET

UNIVERSITY PRESS OF MISSISSIPPI
JACKSON

www.upress.state.ms.us

The University Press of Mississippi is a member of the
Association of American University Presses.

Photographs courtesy of Marcia Gaudet unless otherwise
noted

12 11 10 09 08 07 06 05 04   4 3 2 1

∞

Library of Congress Cataloging-in-Publication Data

Gaudet, Marcia G.
  Carville : remembering leprosy in America / Marcia
Gaudet.
    p. cm.
  Includes bibliographical references and index.
  ISBN 1-57806-693-X (cloth : alk. paper)
  1. National Hansen's Disease Programs Center (U.S.)—
History. 2. Leprosy—United States—Carville—History.
I. Title.
  RA644.L3G38 2004
  362.196'998'00976344—dc22   2004008952

British Library Cataloging-in-Publication Data available

For Irby

Contents

Foreword

Growing up, my daddy convinced me that Carville, Louisiana, was the best place in the entire world. He always made sure I remembered that we had the best climate, the best people, the best family, the best soil, the best peaches—the best everything. I wore my last name with pride—pride that three generations of Carvilles, going back to my great-grandmother Octavia Duhon, provided our town with its postmaster, and then with its name. "Of any place that you could live in the world," my daddy would tell me, "you're living right here in Carville, Louisiana."

Of course, there was another population in Carville, Louisiana. That was the folks at the Gillis W. Long Hansen's Disease Center. From 1894 until 1999, Carville was the home of the only in-patient hospital in the continental United States for the treatment of Hansen's disease, the condition historically called leprosy.

The people who lived at the Center were the last people in America to be formally and legally banished from society because of an illness.

Even though the condition that brought these people to Carville was devastating, the stories that came out of the Center were inspirational.

Through the gates of the Center came ravaged and diseased bodies, broken spirits, people stripped of all dignity and hope. A lot of them had been subjected to the most vile and worst forms of humiliation, degradation, and outright stupidity that a society can heap on people it fears, and things it doesn't understand.

But once inside those gates, people began to gain strength, to heal, to find dignity and hope, and in many cases, love.

Meanwhile, the dedicated physicians and researchers were also finding things—like the sulfone drugs and the multidrug treatment that today allow millions of people with Hansen's to lead a near normal life.

And so, as I grew older, I was able to add another piece of evidence to my daddy's claim that Carville was the best place in the world, and that is because our little town in southern Louisiana became a model for the world, a place of hope, progress, and tolerance.

—JAMES CARVILLE
April 2, 2004

Preface

As a native of Louisiana, I first became aware of Carville and its people in association with election returns (always a colorful topic in this state). Carville is both the name of a small village along the Mississippi River in southern Louisiana and the popular designation or euphemism for a facility established near the village in the late nineteenth century for the isolation and care of leprosy patients. After Carville patients obtained the right to register and vote in 1946, the hospital had its own election precinct. On Election Day, the Carville precinct closed at 4:00 P.M., earlier than any other precinct and usually after all registered voters had voted. The results of the Carville precinct were the first announced by the media in Louisiana. This was remarkable both because there was usually 100 percent voter turnout and also because the results were announced before other polls closed in Louisiana. Many in Louisiana regarded the Carville vote as an early predictor of election results. This announcement was typically followed in the media by a discussion of Carville and its resident patients.

I grew up in a town along the Mississippi River about fifty miles south of Carville. In 1954, I became further aware of leprosy as a disease and of Carville's role in the humane treatment of this illness when a former patient from Carville, Johnny Harmon, moved to the town of Vacherie (near my hometown) and opened a photography business there. His wife, also a patient at Carville, was a native of Vacherie. Though former patients who were released from Carville at that time were encouraged to be open about their illness with the belief that outsiders would accept them, the experience of the Harmons was a rare instance where a community actually did accept former patients without ostracism. A local physician and his wife, Dr. and Mrs. Stephen Campbell, were among the first to have their family's photographs taken by Harmon. Photographs of Dr. Campbell's five daughters were displayed in the shop window. Harmon established a successful business, both as a studio photographer and also as a wedding photographer, photographing over seven hundred weddings in the area, including my brother's wedding to Claire Campbell. My acquaintance with the Harmons' circumstances certainly broadened and enlightened my understanding of people with leprosy—or Hansen's disease, the preferred designation for the illness. When I became interested in collecting and studying narratives and traditions from Carville in

1983, I contacted Johnny Harmon, who still lived in Vacherie at the time. He did not want to talk about his experiences at the time because it would "bring back a lot of bad, painful memories," but his suggestions provided my first introductions at Carville and paved the way for the years of interviews with residents at Carville. In 1993, the Harmons returned to Carville for treatment of various health problems, Mr. Harmon became an outspoken advocate and activist for the dignity and rights of HD patients, and he published his autobiography, *King of the Microbes*. He later talked with me several times about Carville and his experiences as a patient.

Among the many other people who have been important to this study and have helped me in various ways are Dr. Robert Hastings, Julia and Ray Elwood, Esperanza, Rita, Hazel, Billy, Mary Ruth, Louis Boudreaux, Betty Martin, Sister Laura Stricker, Sister Francis de Sales, Sister Margaret Brou, Tanya Thomassie, Father Garland Reynolds, Jane Walters, Elizabeth Schexnyder, Leonide Landry Manes, Claire Manes, Christopher Manes, Jeffrey Braverman, James Carville, Charles Stanley, and the National Hansen's Disease Program. My family, friends, and colleagues were supportive of my work at Carville and often fascinated with the stories I recorded. I am grateful to them all.

Parts of three of the chapters below were previously published as journal articles. I want to acknowledge and thank the journals where they were published. An earlier version of "'Through the Hole in the Fence': Personal Narratives of Absconding From Carville" first appeared in *Fabula* 29 (1988): 354–64. An earlier version of "Telling It Slant: Personal Narratives, Tall Tales, and the Reality of Leprosy" first appeared in *Western Folklore* 49 (1990): 191–207. An earlier version of "The World Downside Up: Mardi Gras at Carville" first appeared in *Journal of American Folklore* 111 (1998): 23–38.

In this book, I look at the memories, narratives, and traditions of former residents of Carville as well as the cultural context the residents had to negotiate. People's most vivid remembrances about what happened to them and their feelings about what happened tend to be clustered around significant events, and their personal narratives reflect this. This study is not intended as a complete history of Carville, nor can it re-create the everyday lives of the residents. Rather, it focuses on memory—what and how Carville residents remember. Their narratives and traditions are vehicles for us to understand something about what they remember about their life experience and how they conceptualize and reconstruct it. The book looks through the prism of memory at how Carville residents dealt with their quest for identity and survival with dignity in spite of their illness. What comes across to the rest of us—through their memories, narratives, traditions, and celebrations—is their humanity. They are *people* who not only survived under difficult conditions but who prevail in the sharing of their memories and stories, connecting us to their humanity.

Carville

To say that Carville is just a place about Hansen's disease would be like saying that Moby Dick *was just a tale about a whale.*

—JAMES CARVILLE
Carville Centennial Speech, 1994

{1} Carville, Leprosy, and Real People

AN INTRODUCTION TO A CULTURE APART

We tell stories because, in order to cope with the present and to face the future, we have to create the past, both as time and space, through narrating it.

—W. F. H. NICOLAISEN

Carville, Louisiana, has been associated with the care and treatment of leprosy patients for over a century. From 1894 to 1999, it was the site of the only in-patient hospital in the continental United States for the treatment of Hansen's disease, the preferred designation for the disease historically called leprosy. Until the 1960s, patients diagnosed in the United States were legally quarantined at Carville. Many never left.

The story of Carville and the patients who were exiled there—for treatment and for separation from the rest of society—is a story of survival and a quest for dignity. It is the story of the place itself and of its former residents who, against many odds, were able to survive the devastating assault that the diagnosis of leprosy brought to their personal identity. When patients entered Carville, they typically left everything behind, including their identities, their legal names, and their hopes for the future.

Of all illnesses, leprosy is probably the one historically most burdened with meanings. Those meanings can range from judgmental and stigmatizing to metaphorical and humorous. Susan Sontag refers to leprosy as "one of the most meaning-laden of diseases" (1989: 92). Like other "meaning-laden" diseases, such as AIDS, it was both a serious illness and a moralistic marker.

In the late nineteenth and early twentieth centuries, the highest incidence of leprosy in the United States was in southern Louisiana. To the Cajuns and Creoles in Louisiana, leprosy was *la maladie que tu nommes pas* (the disease you do not name). A person with a suspected case of leprosy was sometimes hidden and protected by the family. Others were banished by their families when their leprosy was diagnosed. By the mid-1840s, isolation had become an accepted practice in the United States for dealing with leprosy patients. Fear of leprosy was an unquestioned physical reality in Western culture, an accepted fiction based on biblical associations with "lepers."

In speaking of the reaction to cancer as a "demonic enemy" Sontag says in *Illness as Metaphor*, "Any disease that is treated as a mystery and acutely enough feared will be felt to be morally, if not literally, contagious" (1978: 6). She further says: "Leprosy in its heyday aroused a similarly disproportionate sense of horror. In the Middle Ages, the leper was a social text in which corruption was made visible; an exemplum, an emblem of decay. Nothing is more punitive than to give a disease a meaning—that meaning being invariably a moralistic one. Any important disease whose causality is murky, and for which treatment is ineffectual, tends to be awash with significance" (1978: 58).

Untreated leprosy is a serious illness, a disease "written on the skin." As Sander Gilman points out, "all illnesses written on the skin, following the medieval understanding of leprosy as a sexually transmitted disease, are always understood as deforming but also as making one's stigma visible" (Gilman 1988: 76). At least some of the beliefs, laws, and practices from medieval times in regard to leprosy[1] were still haunting patients in the nineteenth century and the first half of the twentieth century. The fear of leprosy in the United States led to the isolation of its victims and eventually to the establishment of Carville.

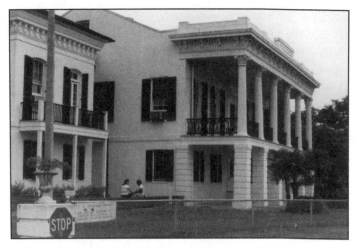

Indian Camp Plantation House. Courtesy of National Hansen's Disease Program.

Carville, as the center was typically called, was established in 1894, a time when leprosy was endemic in certain areas of Louisiana, on a site leased by the Louisiana legislature. It occupied the abandoned slave cabins and plantation home of Indian Camp Plantation, a 395-acre plantation located along the banks of the Mississippi River in Iberville Parish, between New Orleans and Baton Rouge. The action of the legislature to establish a place for both the isolation and humane care of leprosy patients was spurred by New Orleans physician Dr. Isadore Dyer, a dermatologist at Tulane Medical School, who was aware of leprosy cases in New Orleans. Dr. Dyer's efforts were assisted by the New Orleans *Picayune* reporter John Smith Kendall, whose newspaper articles called attention to the plight of leprosy patients in New Orleans.

Leprosy was probably brought to the American continents by early European explorers and settlers and later by enslaved Africans from West Africa (Trautman 1985). In Louisiana, leprosy was reported to have existed under early French and Spanish rule and is thought to have been present in New Orleans in the early eighteenth century. Leprosy reached serious proportions in New Orleans in the early 1780s. The governor, Don Esteban Rodriguez Miro, recommended the building of a "leper" hospital. It was built on Metairie Ridge in 1785, largely funded by the generosity of Don Andrés Almonester, who also funded the new Charity Hospital in New Orleans, completed in 1786. The area came to be known as "La Terre des Lepreux," or "Lepers' Land." By the end of the Spanish period at the beginning of the nineteenth century, the disease was believed to have almost disappeared from Louisiana. There were, however, records of leprosy patients in Charity Hospital in New Orleans at various times throughout the nineteenth century.

Leprosy is also known to have existed among the French in New Brunswick, Canada, as early as 1815 (Stanley 1982, Stanley-Blackwell 1988 and 1993), suggesting a possible connection with leprosy cases among

Acadians in Louisiana. In 1872, Dr. W. G. Kibbe sent a patient from Abbeville in Vermilion Parish to New Orleans to be examined, and the patient was diagnosed with leprosy. Five years later, Dr. Kibbe had seven more patients with leprosy in and around Abbeville (Gussow 1989: 45). In 1880, twelve cases of leprosy were reported in Thibodaux, in Lafourche Parish, about forty miles from New Orleans (Gussow 1989: 48–50). In 1888, more than fifty cases of leprosy were reported in New Orleans, and the *New Orleans Medical and Surgical Journal* recommended the establishment of a separate, new hospital for leprosy patients (Salvaggio 1992: 96). These circumstances led to the actions of Dr. Isadore Dyer and the newspaper reports in the *Picayune* by Kendall in 1894.

Dr. Dyer, with the support of the state legislature, leased Indian Camp Plantation for a five-year term, until he could find a more suitable location closer to New Orleans. The first seven patients arrived at Carville from New Orleans in the middle of the night on December 1, 1894, by barge on the Mississippi River. In April 1896, four Catholic nuns from the Daughters of Charity of St. Vincent de Paul came from Maryland to care for the patients. One of the nuns, Sister Beatrice Hart, was in charge, and the patient population had grown to thirty-one.[2] In 1905, Indian Camp Plantation (originally a Houma Indian village site) was purchased by the state of Louisiana and became the Louisiana

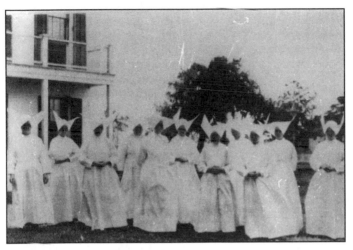

Sisters of Charity (Daughters of Charity of St. Vincent de Paul). Courtesy of National Hansen's Disease Program.

State Home for Lepers. It continued to be run by the Daughters of Charity, who would remain there for over a century. In 1921, it was purchased by the United States government and became the United States Public Health Service Marine Hospital No. 66, known as the National Leprosarium. The need for the U.S. government to establish a National Leprosarium at Carville was given publicity by John Early, a patient from Carville who testified before Congress in 1916. John Ruskin Early, a native of North Carolina, brought national attention to the plight of victims of this disease after he was "charged with a case of leprosy" in 1909 and became notorious for calling attention to his violations of quarantine.³ Later, the name of the Carville hospital was changed from the National Leprosarium to the National Hansen's Disease Center. From 1921 until about 1960, most newly diagnosed patients in the continental United States were required to go to Carville. In 1984 it became the Gillis W. Long National Hansen's Disease Center, named for the Louisiana congressman who supported the wishes of patients by sponsoring a bill to keep the hospital open long after there was any clear medical or fiscal justification for doing so.

In the late nineteenth and early twentieth centuries, leprosy was endemic in parts of Louisiana, Texas, Florida, and New York. There were isolated cases in other areas of the United States as well. Though Massachusetts had also established a state leprosarium in 1905 on Penikese Island in Buzzards Bay, it was closed in 1921 when the thirteen remaining patients were moved to Carville—and the buildings, as well as the boxcar in which they were transported to Louisiana, were burned. There was also a settlement for leprosy patients in San Francisco from about 1850 to 1922. The Kalaupapa settlement for the care of leprosy patients on the island of Molokai in Hawaii was well known internationally because of Father Damien, the Catholic priest who cared for leprosy patients and contracted the disease himself.

An unfortunate result of his fame was reinforcement of fears of leprosy as a highly contagious disease. Louisiana has a somewhat similar case with Father Charles Boglioli, a Catholic priest from Italy who served as chaplain at Charity Hospital in New Orleans beginning in 1866. He attended to the religious needs of several patients with leprosy, and he began to manifest signs of the disease in 1876 or 1877 when he was in his early sixties (Gussow 1989: 50–55). This was almost twenty years before Carville was opened, and there is no record that he was ever at Carville. It is worthwhile to note that no worker, staff member, or visitor in the history of the leprosarium at Carville ever contracted leprosy, and there were daily tours of the center for over sixty years.

Hansen's disease (HD) or leprosy is a disease of the peripheral nerves that also affects the skin. It is probably the least infectious of any communicable disease, and about 95 percent of people have natural immunity. Since leprosy affects relatively few Americans, it is not perceived as a health problem in the United States. Among the misconceptions about HD is that there is a sudden loss of limbs or terrible deformity. This was partially true before there was successful drug treatment, because untreated HD causes nerve damage that can result in loss of feeling, loss of muscle control, and skin lesions. With anesthesia (loss of feeling) in the limbs and face, patients would often injure themselves without realizing it, and this caused some of the deformities. For more than fifty years, a person with HD who is under drug therapy will show no signs of the disease and will certainly not have any body parts simply "fall off" (see Gussow 1979).

Information about Hansen's disease is certainly readily available, most notably from the National Hansen's Disease Program now located in Baton Rouge, Louisiana (website: http://bphc.hrsa.gov/nhdp/default .htm), or through the Global Project on the History of Leprosy, an initiative of the International Leprosy Association (with Nippon Foundation funds through WHO) and the Wellcome Unit For the History of Medicine at Oxford University (website: www.leprosyhistory.org/ english/englishhome.htm). This wealth of information, however, can be confusing because there is still some uncertainty about the transmission, susceptibility, and genetic connection of the disease.

Publications by former directors of the National Hansen's Disease Center at Carville (see especially Trautman and Jacobson) also provide information on the disease, its probable route of transmission, and its physical effects on a patient before and after treatment. Trautman points out that HD exists in almost every country in the world, including the United States, and notes, "Every race is affected by the disease . . . except that, to our knowledge, the disease has never been reported in a full-blooded American Indian" (Trautman 1989). The disease is caused by *Mycobacterium leprae*, but most people have natural immunity to this bacterium. Dr. Gerhard Armauer Hansen was the Norwegian physician who discovered the leprosy bacillus in 1873, a time when leprosy was endemic in Norway. The long incubation period for the disease added to the mystery of its transmission. The period of incubation may be as little as three to five years in susceptible people, but it is believed that it may be as long as twenty years in some cases.

Though it was long suspected that there was some genetic susceptibility to HD, it was not until 2001 that the leprosy genome was decoded and a definite link was identified—a specific genome in 5 percent of people that failed to give them natural immunity. Susceptibility to HD was narrowed down to a specific stretch of DNA, determining that contracting leprosy is impossible without a genetically determined immune deficiency.[4] Thus, though the disease is not hereditary, a genetic susceptibility to the disease may be inherited. Most studies show that men are twice as susceptible as women. Though HD is often believed to be more prevalent in tropical climates, it has also been endemic in very cold climates such as Norway. The mode of transmission is still uncertain, though transmission through respiratory or skin-to-skin contact seems most likely. Since HD or leprosy is a disease of the skin and sensory nerves, untreated HD can result in loss of sensation and deformity, particularly from injuries resulting from loss of feeling in hands and feet. According to Jacobson, a diagnosis of HD "should be considered in any patient with sensory loss and skin lesions" (1990: 1627). There are two majors types of HD, lepromatous and tuberculoid, with a third type, borderline, with characteristics of the two major types. Tuberculoid is the milder form, with fewer effects and symptoms even if untreated. Multidrug therapy (MDT) is used today to quickly arrest the disease and its effects.

Untreated HD can be a physically devastating disease that can lead to severe nerve damage, sensory loss, and disfiguration. Since the 1940s, the disease has been controlled with drug therapy, and most Hansen's disease (HD) patients in the United States are now treated by private physicians or at regional Public Health Service—supported HD outpatient clinics. These are located in cities throughout the United States, including New York, Boston, Los Angeles, San Diego, Chicago, Miami, Seattle, and Honolulu. Treatment now renders it almost immediately noncommunicable, though it is only minimally communicable at any time after prolonged contact with an active case. There are about six thousand diagnosed cases of Hansen's disease in the United States and an estimated four thousand undiagnosed cases. Only about six hundred of these are in need of active medical treatment at any one time. The discovery in 1971 that nine-banded armadillos could be infected with the leprosy bacillus, and therefore could be used as test animals, enabled research that led to successful treatment and ultimately a cure for leprosy. Armadillos in the wild are now believed to have about a 5 percent rate of naturally occurring infection with the leprosy bacillus (based on studies in Texas and Louisiana). It is believed to be the only animal susceptible to leprosy. The armadillo became the symbol of leprosy research and, perhaps ironically, also the symbol on Carville Mardi Gras doubloons, the aluminum coins tossed or thrown to spectators during Mardi Gras parades.[5]

Though leprosy is an ancient disease, the disease as we know it today is not believed to be the same as biblical leprosy. In *Some Questions Commonly Asked About Hansen's Disease. . . . and Some Concise Answers*, a book that was published at Carville for newly diagnosed patients, Dr. John Trautman wrote: "The description of 'leprosy' which is found in Leviticus is definitely not the same as the disease known today as leprosy or Hansen's disease. . . . Apparently what was being described in the Bible was a ritual Hebrew 'uncleanliness,' not a human disease of skin and nerves" (n.d.: 8). Trautman also writes: "The first thing we'd like to do is simply to assure you that, rumors and stories aside, Hansen's disease is essentially a disease like any other" (n.d., 2). While this may be true from a medical point of view, HD patients historically were certainly not treated like patients of any other disease by society in general or by the government.

Louisiana's establishment of an institution for the humane care and treatment of leprosy patients in 1894 resulted in Carville's eventually becoming an international medical research center for leprosy, credited with the eventual discovery of a cure.[6] For leprosy patients in the early twentieth century, however, admittance to the institution at Carville was tantamount to imprisonment. Because leprosy patients in the United States were subject to legal quarantine for more than half of the twentieth century, they were "sentenced" by law in most states to exile in Carville. It was not a real quarantine since patients were regularly given passes to visit their families, and many left illegally "through the hole in the fence." The diagnosis of leprosy, however, was a traumatic and life-altering shock.[7] New patients at Carville not only took on sudden stigmatization, but they were also likely to lose much of their former identities, including their names. While being admitted to Carville, patients were encouraged to hide their true identities. Often not even the staff knew their real

names. No identification papers were necessary to enter
and often even the hometown was kept secret so the
shame and ostracism would not extend to their families.

Assigning "meanings" to a disease (Sontag 1978 and
1989), as well as representing illness and disease in art,
literature, and popular culture, also contributes to beliefs
and fears attached to disease (Gilman 1988 and 1995).
This has been particularly true with leprosy, evidenced
by the continued metaphorical usage of terms associated
with the disease to denote a person who is shunned or
avoided by others. The persistence of the leprosy stigma
is evident in the fact that most patients kept their diagnosis a secret from all but trusted family and friends
(Gussow and Tracy 1969 and 1971, and Kalisch 1973).
Until the 1980s, all people diagnosed with leprosy in the
United States were assured lifetime care at Carville if
they chose to stay or return. Carville stopped accepting
permanent residents in 1986. Of the approximately three
hundred patients at Carville in the 1980s, many were
international residents of the United States who had no
medical insurance. Most were treated and released.
Another group of about fifty patients were older residents who had entered Carville before there was effective treatment for the disease and when there was still
compulsory isolation, some as early as the 1920s. They
had lived at Carville most of their lives, and they

remained there voluntarily. Some had nowhere else to go, and others did not want to readjust to a world that had once ostracized them.

Since the early 1980s, the federal government has proposed various uses for the Carville complex, including an experiment with the U.S. Bureau of Prisons from 1991 to 1994, when the residents at Carville shared the complex with federal prisoners. Carville was closed as a treatment center for leprosy in 1999, a victim of its own success. The federally owned campus-style hospital complex in Carville was transferred to the State of Louisiana for the purpose of establishing a youth job-training center there, and the medical and research divisions of the National Hansen's Disease Program were moved to Baton Rouge.

Former patients at Carville were the last group of people in America to be formally and legally banished by society because of an illness. They created a culture of their own at Carville. Gussow and Tracy pointed out in 1971: "'Returnees' and those patients who never left have formed a quite stable kind of community, or 'colony,' within the hospital. A kind of 'culture of differentness' has been established" (Gussow and Tracy 1971: 697). For many years this community was a close-knit group with their own holiday celebrations, recreations, traditions, stories, and legends. After legal quarantine ended, many older patients remained there at least partly by choice. Similar to other elderly groups who

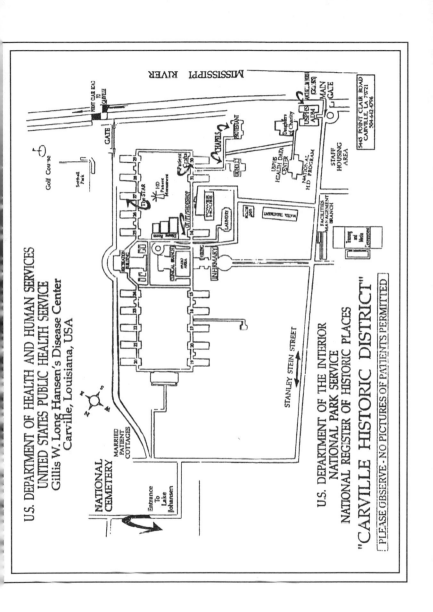

have formed communities, particularly those with "survivor's" vitality (See Myerhoff 1979), their customs, celebrations, and personal narratives enhanced the quality of their lives and gave them additional, more meaningful bonds. They were part of a true folk community at Carville—isolated from the rest of the world with their own traditions, celebrations, stories, and views of the outside world.

The Hansen's Disease Center at Carville had many of the marks and establishments of a typical rural Louisiana community, including an infirmary, a school, a bank, a store, a library, two churches, a bar, a jail, a golf course, a lake for boating and fishing, and a cemetery. The patients had holiday celebrations, such as Mardi Gras balls and parades, a softball team that played other teams in the River League, and an active social club. Unlike other communities, however, the shared identity of Carville residents was based on their shared medical diagnosis, Hansen's disease—or leprosy. They were victims of a mildly infectious disease that was surrounded by mystery and often irrational fear. The HD community at Carville differed as well from others in rural Louisiana in the early twentieth century in how it dealt with race. It was a highly unusual institution located in the American South, a region with legal segregation of the races. While the isolation and separation of leprosy patients may have had similar roots in the kinds of

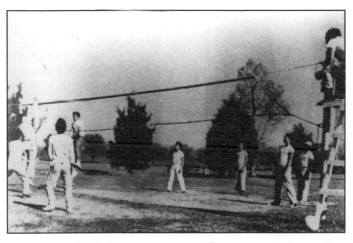

Patients' volleyball game, ca. 1940. Courtesy of National Hansen's Disease Program.

ignorance and fears that foster other exclusionary practices, such as racial segregation, patients at Carville were not further stigmatized within their community because of race. This can probably be attributed both to the influence of the Daughters of Charity and to the fact that after 1921, Carville was under federal rather than state law. Though patients were segregated by gender in the early days of the center, there is little evidence at any attempts at racial segregation. An illustration of the Carville classroom in a 1948 edition of *The Star* shows black and white students together. The caption reads, "Real Golden Rule Days—A rare sight in the Deep South—a school without a color line. Bound together by mutual affliction, these children study and play without prejudice" (National Leprosarium 1948: 13). Photographs of the baseball team, school classroom, Boy Scout troop, dances, picnics, fishing rodeos, clubs, choirs, socials, and so forth throughout the twentieth century indicate a multicultural and multiracial community, separated from the outside world but not from each other.[8]

Any culture that is isolated, for whatever reason, is likely to be rich in traditional folkloric material—narratives, customs, rituals, artifacts, and so forth—and this was especially true of the community at Carville. Patients at Carville used these traditional resources, along with personal and political agency, to help shape their own self-understanding, to maintain some dignity and control over their lives, and to negotiate their relationship with the outside world. Carville residents not only survived but through their actions, verbal strategies, and self-understanding were often able to see the ironies and absurdities of their situation and to respond with humor, even at times laughing at the society from which they had been banished. Strong will and imagination kept them searching for ways of taking some control of a situation in which, by law, they had little or no control. Their sense of dignity and worth evolved within the context of their efforts to overcome public perception and treatment.

Patients used discursive practices and performances to reestablish and maintain their sense of identity and dignity. They used their own customs and traditions to maintain their sense of community. They used personal narratives to empower themselves and in some cases to politicize their quest for human and civil rights. There was an ongoing push to be treated as human beings—to assert their own *dignity*, whether others recognized it or not.

In *Illness and Culture in the Postmodern Age*, David Morris says:

> Illness threatens to undo our sense of who we are. Its darkest power lies in showing us a picture of ourselves—false, damaged, unreliable, and inescapably mortal—that we desperately do not want to see. A serious and protracted illness constitutes an immersion in an alien reality where almost everything changes. At its most dire, it can wreck the body, unstring the mind, and paralyze the emotions, plunging entire families into bankruptcy and chaos. Fortunately, most illnesses do not last long enough to create a permanent schism in our sense of self or to change our vision of the world. (Morris 1998: 22)

Morris's description of serious illness accurately portrays what seems to have been the initial response of people diagnosed with HD. Unlike most other serious illnesses, for much of history HD did not kill, but it lasted for what was often a very long lifetime of isolation and disfigurement. Leprosy not only stigmatized, it transformed basic identity. Unlike any other illness, this disease branded its victims with its name. One became a "leper" with all the judgment-laden associations from the Bible, from literature, and from popular culture.

HD patients at Carville provide a study of how people in twentieth-century America, caught in the circumstances of a "medieval" illness, sought to regain their sense of self, their sense of worth, and a sense of their own dignity. In the cultural context they had to negotiate, narratives of trauma, ostracism, and ultimate survival later served to empower patients. The recurring humor in these Carville stories is striking. However despairing the circumstances, most of the narrators eventually saw sources of laughter in their situation, calling to mind Anatole Broyard's statement about his own life-threatening sickness: "Illness is not all tragedy. . . . Much of it is funny" (1992: 46). Through their memory and narratives, we see their very human quest for identity and their survival with dignity and grace.

{2} "An Exile in My Own Country"

THE UNSPEAKABLE TRAUMA OF ENTERING CARVILLE

At ten o'clock on that Sunday morning, March 1, 1931, I became an exile in my own country.

—STANLEY STEIN
Alone No Longer

A diagnosis of leprosy was inevitably traumatic. Such a diagnosis was usually totally unexpected as well. Even when the diagnosis was not a complete surprise (because of the knowledge that other family members had the disease), it was still devastating. In such cases, the patients had already witnessed the trauma, knew something of what awaited them, and may have lived in dread of their own diagnosis. In addition, the diagnosis was usually followed either by an attempt to conceal the nature of the disease if possible or the necessity for virtual "exile" to Carville. New patients at Carville not only took on sudden stigmatization but also were likely to lose much of their former identities, including their names. Patients being admitted to Carville were encouraged to hide their true identities. Often not even the staff knew their real names. No identification papers were necessary to enter, and even the hometown was kept secret so the shame and ostracism would not extend to their families. As Gussow and Tracy point out, "Diagnosis of leprosy with or without concomitant hospitalization, signals a sudden, radical, undesired, and unanticipated transformation of the patient's life program" (1968: 319).

For all Hansen's disease patients, there was an initial, devastating trauma—being told that they had leprosy and would be quarantined at Carville. In order to have some control over their own existence, they first had to come to terms with what it meant to suffer from Hansen's disease in the twentieth century. Some had to overcome their own self-aversion as "lepers" and to arrive at some understanding of how this most meaning-laden of diseases differed from other diseases because of the historical stigma of leprosy rooted in the Bible.

For many former Carville patients, their memories were (and are) what Roberta Culbertson calls "embodied memory"—memory that is bodily, a sense memory (1995: 174–75).[1] In leprosy or any trauma that manifests itself daily in scars or bodily signs, the inability to conceal the bodily memory is likely to complicate traditional survival strategies and add social traumas to the medical trauma. Weaving the traumatic threads into a cohesive narrative is a way of dealing with the trauma, particularly in a disease where the social construction or common (albeit erroneous) understanding is one of the body literally falling apart.

For those who left Carville for a time, their very survival on the outside depended upon their not giving voice to those memories. In assuming a new identity, they had to subvert the need to speak, to give narrative form to the trauma of being diagnosed with leprosy, torn from family and friends, sent to Carville, and advised to change their names—to protect their families. In order to "pass" as "healthy" or normal on the outside they had to hide their illness from employers, friends, and sometimes even their own children. They not only had to hide their diagnosis and their time spent at Carville but often had to silence memories of the initial trauma as well as lost years of their lives.

This chapter will focus on how former patients at Carville remember the trauma of being diagnosed with leprosy, how they chose to voice those memories in personal narrative, and how they were able to reconstruct their own identities through knowledge, understanding, and the assertion of personal agency. Having survived an unspeakable trauma, they were empowered to give voice to their memories.

The personal narratives and life writings of former Carville patients reflect this trauma and devastation. Stanley Stein describes his admittance to Carville in his 1963 autobiography, *Alone No Longer*: "I had arrived at U.S. Marine Hospital No. 66, Carville, Louisiana, then as now, the only institution in the continental United States devoted exclusively to the treatment of leprosy. At ten o'clock on that Sunday morning, March 1, 1931, I became an exile in my own country" (4). Stein came to Carville from Boerne, Texas, where he was a pharmacist. His family was German and Jewish, and they knew of no one else in the family who had the disease. He was an educated person who loved music and the arts, but like other patients he became a number at Carville: "Henceforth I would always be No. 746, a number identified not only with my case history but with everything I would do at Carville for the next third of a century. . . . I was sinking into the quagmire of anonymity which society reserves for the victims of leprosy, mental illness, or crime. We were no more entitled to individuality than a convict in a penitentiary" (11). He describes the shock of entering Carville and the horror of seeing the "grotesque masks" of the advanced cases. His first night at Carville was terrifying and overpowering. The next morning was worse:

> I was not completely submerged, however, until a doctor stuck his head into the Record Room and administered the coup de grace. In the months ahead we were to become friends, but at that moment I hated him with all my heart, for he was destroying the last link to my old life.
>
> "Morning, Sister Laura. . . . New patient, I see. What name is he taking?"
>
> Another name? What was wrong with my own name? Did I have to hide under an alias like a hunted criminal? Could I keep nothing of my old life to clothe my naked ego?
>
> "Have you decided on your new name, young man?" Sister Laura asked sweetly.
>
> I shook my head. I was too crushed to speak. (11)

Stein says, "Leprosy was not just a disease—it was a stigma, a disgrace, a visitation from on high, a punishment for some dreadful sin" (21). He chose the alias Stanley Stein, giving up his real name, Maurice Levyson.

Betty Parker Martin came to Carville from New Orleans in January 1928, shortly after her diagnosis of leprosy in December 1927. She was nineteen years old and recently

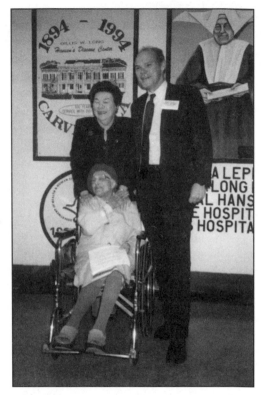

Betty Martin, Lucille (Nippy) Carville, and James Carville, Carville Centennial Celebration, 1994. James Carville was the keynote speaker for the celebration, and his mother, Nippy Carville, was a member of the Centennial Advisory Board. The town of Carville was named for its postmaster, Louis Arthur Carville, the grandfather of James Carville. Courtesy of National Hansen's Disease Program.

engaged to a medical student. Her 1950 best-selling autobiography, *Miracle at Carville*, tells the story of life in the leprosarium, her marriage to another patient, their life after release, and the necessity for concealing their disease and their real names. Betty and Harry Martin, a former LSU football player, returned to Carville in 1990 because of Mr. Martin's health, after having lived on the "outside" for almost fifty years.

In *Miracle at Carville*, Betty Martin describes the devastation not only to herself but to her whole family when her illness was diagnosed, saying that her father "wept for two days and nights" (3). She describes her own response to the news as at first disbelief and shock. Then she says: "As shock gave way to realization every nerve and muscle in my body leapt and twitched; there was no reason in me, I was just a shivering bundle of fear. If I had been told I would die on the morrow I doubt if the shock would have been so great, in fact death would have seemed simple by comparison. When one died, all was over, but I had to go on living and fighting a self violated in a mysterious fashion by an insidious disease" (9). She also indicates in her book that she had no clue as to how she had contracted the disease at such a young age. She says, "Nineteen. I searched those years and I search them still, finding nothing in them but the purest happiness, the sanest, healthiest living. Nowhere along the road, hunt as I might, could I find any indication of a shadowy place where this evil thing, reaching out, had touched me" (13). She describes hearing the words "leper" and "leprosy" applied to her for the first time as a "soul-searing experience" (263).

When Betty entered Carville on January 15, 1928, there were 440 patients there. Photographs show her to be a beautiful young woman. Stanley Stein says in *Alone No Longer*, "I have seen few women, at Carville or elsewhere, as beautiful as Betty Parker who later married handsome Harry Martin and whose moving love story is known to the many thousands who read her *Miracle at Carville*" (109). Upon entering Carville, Betty Parker Martin saw for the first time the disfigurement caused by the disease. A patient came to her room the first night she was there and said to her, "I looked just like you when I came here, and look at me now!" (19). In the 1999 documentary, *Banished: Living with Leprosy*, Betty read from her book. Of her admittance to Carville, she said, "It was horrible." Betty was mercifully spared the worst effects of Hansen's disease, and when she died in June 2002, her face was still unmarked by the disease. However, the trauma to her family was still very real. In planning her funeral in Baton Rouge in June 2002, her brother-in-law reportedly said, "We don't want Carville mentioned at this funeral." Her obituary, using only her real name, made no mention of Betty Martin, and there was no acknowledgment in the media that Betty Martin, author of *Miracle at Carville*, had died. Her family honored her wishes as reflected in the title of her second book, *No One Must Ever Know* (1959).

Johnny Harmon entered Carville on August 2, 1935, at the age of twenty-four. He was forced to leave his hometown of Hankamer, Texas, and the life he had known as a draftsman for the Texas Highway Department. Since his older brother had been diagnosed earlier by a Houston doctor and entered Carville in 1934, his own diagnosis was not a complete surprise to him. The effects were no less traumatic. In a 1998 interview with CNN reporter Charles Zewe, Harmon said, "The bottom seems to fall out, and you know darn well you've passed through a door that you're never going to come back out of." In Harmon's memoir, *King of the Microbes* (1999), he describes his family's response to his brother Elmo's diagnosis: "It took Dr. Michael only a matter of minutes to give us the tragic news. He wrote something on a piece of paper and handed it to my father. A word as old as time itself. A word that scares the living daylights out of almost everyone. LEPROSY" (5). Later, he says, "In the Fall and Winter of 34, I noticed that the little finger of my left hand had lost sensation. . . . By then I knew that my life as a normal person was over" (18). Johnny's case was relatively mild, and he was released in 1938. He lived in Beaumont until he reentered Carville in 1942, Patient No. 1541, because his symptoms had become worse, and he could no longer hide them. His brother Elmo had died in Carville in 1941. Johnny said, "I witnessed every stage of his horrible disfiguring disease when there was no medicine to fight it with" (64). When Johnny reentered, there was effective treatment. In a 1996 interview, Johnny Harmon told me he thought he would be there for life. He said, "It was really frightening when I came in." Eventually he became the official photographer for *The Star*, the publication that began as a mimeographed patient newsletter and eventually became an internationally distributed publication to "promote an educated public opinion of Hansen's disease." Harmon's cartoons as well as his photographs were published in *The Star* under his Carville alias, J. P. Harris. In the last few years of his life, Johnny became somewhat of a celebrity. CNN interviewed him, and *People* magazine as well as other national publications published articles about him. He also appeared in three documentaries on Carville. When he died in September 2002, the *New Orleans Times-Picayune* published a major article about and a photograph of him (Pope B-5). Johnny, of course, had openly acknowledged his illness and was the rare HD patient who did become a kind of hero in his community. He also became a spokesperson for educating the public about Hansen's disease and for promoting the dignity and rights of HD patients. Before Johnny died, he said in an interview, "They changed the name, but we haven't changed the disease. People are still afraid of us . . . and I want them to know that it's not contagious, and people are not lepers, they're people." (Pope B-5). He also said, "God's been good to me, in spite of the disease . . . You may think I'm crazy, but I think I've lived a fuller life because I've had the disease because I've met all kinds of people that I wouldn't have met before" (Pope B-5).

Stanley Stein, Betty Martin, and Johnny Harmon were, of course, extraordinary people as well as HD patients. All three wrote and published their life stories, becoming spokespersons for the disease. While the very earliest patients were silenced and many never were heard, later patients empowered themselves to speak.[2] While Carville may have been a "secret place" at one time, particularly for those whose families deserted them—and many were totally silenced, their voices never to be heard—the people who wrote their memoirs and those I interviewed were *not* silent. In fact, they were quite outspoken. They willingly spoke through *The Star* (reaching a wide audience), through letters,[3] through interviews, and through legal action.

While patients told their stories in some interviews, there was still the need to be careful, and clearly the memory of the traumatic experience of coming to Carville was a painful one. Regarding memories of their diagnosis, Carville residents told Mississippi writer Barry Hannah in 1995 that coming to Carville made them "too devastated" to remember their reactions or details from the experience. Hannah says in an article in *Oxford American*: "It is remarkable that when I asked patient after patient whether they had anger—at God, luck, fate—when they first heard their diagnosis, all of them replied no. The desolation was so complete they could not recall another emotion" (47). Many of the residents, however, did remember quite vividly their diagnosis and introduction to Carville. They recorded these memories in memoirs and told their stories to me and to many others who interviewed them. There were stories clustered around arrival at Carville, as well as escaping from Carville, "putting on" outsiders, and participating in traditions such as the annual Mardi Gras celebration.

What is even more remarkable is how patients who came to Carville were able to construct new identities for themselves. What becomes evident is that these people eventually came to terms with their diagnosis, and they were able to establish a life for themselves, either in Carville or on the "outside." Many became spokespersons for the disease—demanding collectively that their voices be heard (at least by the United States government) and their basic rights restored.

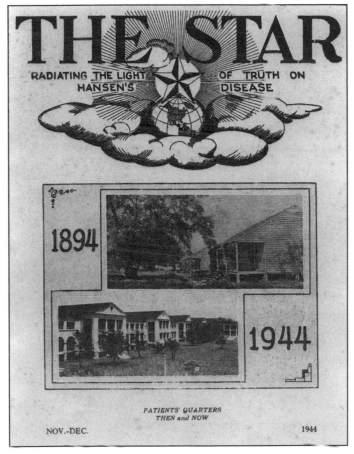

Cover of the first printed issue of The Star, *1944. Courtesy of National Hansen's Disease Program.*

Stanley Stein is credited with developing patients' rights coalitions, exerting influence to obtain rights for the patients, including the rights to vote and to marry. One of his major accomplishments was to establish a newsletter for patients, which he called *The Sixty-Six Star*, a mimeographed sheet that he edited and distributed. The first issue was dated May 16, 1931. On June 10, 1944, the first printed edition of *The Star* was published, primarily a patients' magazine but destined to become an international publication on Hansen's disease. The goal of the publication was stated in the motto, "Radiating the Light of Truth on Hansen's Disease." Stanley Stein says in *Alone No Longer*, "It is not what we have lost that matters most, but what we chose to do with what we have left." This choice to move on, to recognize the devastation of their diagnosis but to find a way to make a life for themselves is evident in the personal narratives of several of the former Carville patients I interviewed, starting in 1983 and continuing through 2002. In interviewing Carville residents, I was interested in why those particular things and occasions were memorable to them, what meanings those memories had for them, why certain ones got memorialized into stories, how they were transmitted, and what purposes they served.

Louis Boudreaux, who served as editor of *The Star* for many years, was from a small town across the Mississippi River and about fifteen miles south of Carville. In a 1983

interview, he told me about the trauma of learning
that he had leprosy. When I asked him if he had
changed his name, he responded:

> Yes, because we were encouraged to do that . . . when I
> came here . . . to protect the family. We had to maintain
> the secrecy because lots of times the family suffered
> more than the patients did as a result of the disease.
> My brothers and sisters were put out of school and my
> father had a little business—and his business suffered
> terribly, and he almost went bankrupt. Simply because
> people were afraid . . . And I don't blame them–or I did
> not blame them at that time, because I was just as
> afraid as everyone else when I came to Carville. I knew
> very little or nothing at all, and what I knew was what
> I read in the paper. I was afraid, so I couldn't blame the
> general public. But it's a shame though, that today even
> we have friends far away who have a better understand-
> ing of this disease, than in surrounding areas. We have
> people in Baton Rouge who have never been to this
> place. (Personal interview, 1983)

Louis Boudreaux kept his "Carville name," even as editor of *The Star*. He worked with Stanley Stein as an
assistant, and later became an important force in using
personal experience narratives as well as editorial writing for political purposes.

The importance of secrecy from the early days is
evident in this excerpt from a letter written by the first

four Sisters of Charity to their superiors in Emmitsburg, Maryland: "The lepers made and still make it a point to keep secret their names and their family history. This but proves the horror with which the disease is regarded. The leper dies when he enters the institution. He does not forget, but he is a forgotten man" (Elwood 1996: 51).

Hazel, a native of St. Louis, was eighty-five years old when I talked with her in 1983. She had first come to Carville in 1922, the divorced mother of a six-month-old daughter. She had been a discharged patient since 1946, but she came back to Carville in 1969 because of cataracts. Hazel said that when the doctor in St. Louis first diagnosed her disease, he put her in isolation in a hospital, but he did not immediately tell her family what it was. She and her family learned her diagnosis by reading it in the *Globe-Democrat*. The headline the next morning was "Girl Leper Found in St. Louis." She still remembered this experience vividly and could describe it in detail:

> Well, I had lots of infections. And, I'd show them to my mother, and say, "Look, my whole skin is bleeding, and I don't feel it." And I didn't feel a thing. And then my mother would take me to the doctor, and he'd look at it, and say, "There's nothing wrong with that girl. Just rub it. Poor circulation." And I just kept going—And

then my mother said, "I don't know who to take you to anymore." And then, I got some—what you call "tubercles." And then they'd come out, and you'd put this cream on them, and they'd go away. Then, there was a German doctor. He treated venereal disease. And my mother wouldn't take me to him. And this lady said, "I don't care what–he's a German doctor and he's a very good doctor. I would take her there. . . ." When she took me to this German doctor, and he looked at me and he was checking the reflexes in my knee . . . but he was really seeing if I would scream. And I didn't like the way he was looking at me. So, he said, okay, you come back next week, and he gave me the day. So, my mother was working then, and my daddy was working at night. My mother was working in one of the leading stores in St. Louis, downtown, and she was demonstrating instant cake flour. And I had to go to the doctor. So my daddy said, "Well, I can stay with her [the baby] until about 5 o'clock." So I went to the doctor's office, and his office went into the hall, so I went into one with the reception room, and I waited and I waited. And people would come and people would go. And I said, "Well, this is funny. I sit here. I came here first, and I'm still sitting here." Well, ah, the receptionist said, "Please wait." Then, a doctor came in, and he came in the wrong office—he came in the reception room. And, "Oh," he said, "I'm Dr. Henry. I'm from the Health Department. I came in the wrong office."

And I don't know why—I looked at that man, and I said, "That man is looking for me." I don't know why—if you're sitting in an office, and they're taking everybody else, and let you sit there, wouldn't you have felt the same way?" And then one of the doctors called me, and I dropped my purse—I was so nervous. And them days, you didn't go anywhere without a hat, so I had my hat, and I dropped my hat—cause I was so nervous. So I went in there, and the doctor said, "This is Dr. Henry from the Health Department." And I looked at him, and he said, "Now you go along with him in his car, and he'll take you along to the city hospital." And I said, "My mother and father are waiting for me to come home." So we went down there, and we went to this hall and that hall. And then he said, "You've got to go in this room." And I knew it was an isolation ward. That's where they used to put the smallpox patients there . . . to be quarantined. And I said, "I'm not going in the room. If I go in the room, they're not going to let me come out." "Well you have to go in there." "No, I don't have to do it." And he said, "Well, you have to take some tests." They had a special nurse and a special orderly for me. And they notified my mother at home [that I was in quarantine], and she almost fainted. They didn't tell me at first it was leprosy. They said, "Have you ever been in the Orient?" I said, "No." "You ever been to Chicago?" I said, "No. I never been out of St. Louis in my life." They said, "You ever been with a Chinaman?" I said, "No." I was scared to death of Chinamen. . . . So they didn't tell me anything. On Sunday morning, the *Globe Democrat*, our main paper Sunday morning in St. Louis, they had across the top of the paper, "Girl Leper Found in St. Louis." They didn't tell my family [that it was leprosy]. And my brother went down to get the paper, and he seen it. And they said, "Harry, you got the paper," and he said, "Yea." And he gave it to my mother, and when she read it, she fainted. My brother wanted to go down there and beat that doctor [she laughs]. My brother was eight years older than me, and my father said, "No, you're not going to go down there." My family wanted to come down here with me [to Carville]. I said, "No, you have to stay in St. Louis and take care of my daughter." March 19, 1922. When we came up the road, I said, "What's that hill there?" [Laughs] That was the levee. I came on St. Joseph Day. That was my father's birthday.

. . . When I came down, the government reserved one car. And they hooked it on to the other cars. And they had some patients in Chicago that they picked up, and then they came to St. Louis to pick me up. (Personal interview 1984)

Hazel later went on to say:

And I divorced my husband. His family— those days were different from these days. His family was scared to death, and I knew I was coming here. Well, I thought, this is the end. Because when I came, in those days, you came in, but you couldn't go out that gate, not on a vacation or anything. My people could come visit me . . . I thought, well, I was here and that was it. So I said to my mother and my father, "You raise my baby." But, things changed over the years. Cause then the only way you could leave was with twelve negative tests. (Personal interview 1984)

No children under sixteen were allowed in Carville at that time (except as patients), so Hazel's daughter could not visit her there when she first came to Carville. Though Hazel was from St. Louis, when she left Carville illegally a few years later, she did not return there because she feared she would be found by authorities. She went to Chicago instead, and her mother and daughter joined her in Chicago. Hazel said, "When I went home [the first time, without official leave] she knew about me, since my mother had told her about me, but she didn't know me. She was a little five-year-old child. So, I had to get acquainted with her. I went back [to Carville] when she was nine years old." She didn't tell her daughter what she had or where she was until she was sixteen. Hazel's mother told her that she was in a hospital for a nervous breakdown.

Hazel arrived at Carville one year after the federal government took over the hospital, and made it a National Leprosarium. Until 1921, it had been the Louisiana Leper Home, and most of the patients were from Louisiana at that time. Hazel used to sew and made all of her daughter's clothes. She said, "I always kept busy." She also said, "We had what we called the

'What Cheer' Club. We had a canteen that ran the What Cheer Club. I didn't know how to sew when I came here, so I had to learn. I could make dresses without a pattern. I would look at dresses in McCall's."

Hazel married another Carville patient in 1936. They weren't supposed to leave the state or use public transportation, but they went to Gulfport, Mississippi, to be married because Louisiana required a blood test for a marriage license. She said that people were able to build a meaningful life for themselves and to adjust to the reality of their lives in Carville. She said, "We made our own pleasure. . . . You'd be surprised at how well they do adjust. . . . It isn't so bad, you know." She later added, "They don't call it a leper colony any more. It's time to get away from that. It's a Hansen's Disease Center." Hazel died at Carville in 1985.

Rita was twenty years old when she entered Carville in 1927. She said the only person she knew who had the disease (before she came to Carville) was her uncle's wife. Rita was from a little town in St. John the Baptist Parish called Wallace (now part of Vacherie), about thirty miles south of Carville. Her aunt was from Garyville. Rita was the fourth of ten children and the oldest girl. She was eleven when her mother died, leaving a baby only a few months old, and Rita had the responsibility of caring for the younger children. She found out she had the disease after her boyfriend reported her symptoms to the local physician. When I asked her about her diagnosis and how it was found out, she said:

> Son of a gun of a man—from my boyfriend. It started out that I had a little lesion on my face—like a breaking out, you know. And then, when I went across to see my girlfriend one day, I had no feeling at all. I cut myself on a wire, and I didn't know it. And that's where it started. Me and my girlfriend, we went to visit a relative in Garyville, and we walked by that pond. There was a big rain, and we got soaking wet. And then we had to catch a train to Lutcher. It was my uncle's wife who had it. I got it from her. My boyfriend told the doctor. He wrote a letter to the doctor in Vacherie—Dr. Lionel Waguespack. He [her boyfriend] said he fell in love at first sight. He said he was so much in love with me, he said if anything should ever happen, he would climb a mountaintop [to be with her]. And I felt like writing to him after I came here, and I'd say, "Are you still going to climb the mountaintop?" (Laughter). No, no, no, no. That was the end of his love affair. (Personal interview 1983)

Rita's father and siblings never came to visit her after she came to Carville. Her father brought her to Carville, and she never saw him again until his funeral. Her family told people that she had died, and she herself was told nothing by her father about her diagnosis until she arrived at Carville.

After coming to Carville, Rita went back home to Vacherie only once, for her father's funeral:

> Yes—I went—. I wanted to see my father—before—before I went blind. And my sisters, they wouldn't let me see him—wouldn't let me see him. I never seen my father. I didn't—. They [her nieces] came and get me for the funeral, but I didn't want to go. But my nieces said, "Yes, you're gonna go. You're gonna go, gonna go." They [her sisters] were scared of me, that's why. But my nieces, when they found out I was here, they came. Their Mama [wife of her brother] treated me better than my own sisters. These two nieces . . . Yes, I went to my father's funeral. The sisters still didn't even talk to me, but my sister-in-law. . . . I said when I die, I don't want none of them to come— (Personal interview 1983)

Rita said that her two nieces still visited her at Carville, but their father did not, though he knew where she was. When I asked her what her father had told her brothers and sisters when she left for Carville, she said:

> I don't know, to tell you the truth. But they knew . . . my big brother knew. [At the funeral] my niece said, "You want to see Daddy?" And I said, "Well, here I am. I'm sick, but I'm not dead yet." Because that's what they had told everybody. You know my daddy said I was dead—. I said, "Here I am. Very much alive. Not dead yet." I never heard from them, and I never

> inquired. . . . My sister was a nurse. She wasn't that
> stupid. When I'd write letters, they would hide them.
> They'd burn them right away. My father dropped me
> here, and he never came back. . . . They didn't tell me
> nothing. My father didn't tell me nothing. (Personal
> interview 1984)

Rita later married another patient, a man from Garyville
who was many years older than she. She said, "He was
a nice-looking man." At that time, patients from
Louisiana could have a pass for ten days, and they were
married in Poplarville, Mississippi. When they got back,
her husband was put in the jail ("Not too long. Just to
say they did something"), and she was confined to the
hospital. But they let him come to visit her every day.
They had a cottage of their own at Carville, and they
were neighbors of Stanley Stein, Harry and Betty Martin,
Louis and Kitty Boudreaux, Johnny and Ann Harmon,
and others, including Mary Ruth and Darryl.

Mary Ruth came to Carville in 1939, the same
year that her future husband, Darryl, whom she met
at Carville, entered. Mary was twenty-two. She had
grown up in Texas, and she was living with her mother
and working in San Antonio when she was diagnosed.
Mary did not know that her sister Kitty (who later
married Louis Boudreaux) had been diagnosed with
leprosy earlier and was already at Carville until shortly

before Mary herself came to Carville as a patient. In an interview with me in April 2001, she said:

> I didn't know she was here. I didn't know it until a few months before I came. And when I told my mother about me, and, ah, we were saying the rosary, it was night, about 8 o'clock, and I started crying. I started thinking, "What am I going to do all alone?" And my mother got up and came over to me and said, "What's the matter." So I told her what I had. I hadn't told my mother. Oh, yes, I knew it for about three months and I kept it to myself. Where I worked, you had to get an exam every six months. And I had a big spot right there. That's the way it was. I was taking menus in a hospital, and giving out nourishments, and bringing mail to the patients. I took a blood test. They gave me a blood test, and they thought I had syphilis. And I didn't even know what it was to be with a man. Of course, I didn't tell my mother, because I didn't know what syphilis in Spanish is either [i.e., the Spanish word for syphilis]. My mother spoke English very little. She spoke Spanish and French. She was from Mexico, but her mother was from France. [When I told her what I had] that's when she told me my sister was here. Ah! I thought she was in New Orleans studying. I thought she was going to college. So the next day, I got on the bus. I went to see Dr. Woods, and I told him everything, what my mother told me and all. He said, "Now you're gonna like Carville." I don't know if I thought about it when he told me, or if I started thinking about it when I got here.

I don't know. I was lonesome, even though my sister was here. And, ah, how many years did I have to stay here? So, I asked my sister, "How long do you have to stay?" I didn't use the word "discharged" because I didn't know it [laughter]. [The doctor in San Antonio had told her she would have to stay three or four years.] I said, "That's a long time." But you know what, that was my happiest years, cause I found my honey [laughter]. We didn't get married until 1946. [Kitty and Louis got married in November 1945.] (Personal interview 2001)

By the late 1950s, most states no longer had legal quarantine of patients with HD. Treatment for most patients, however, was available only at Carville. Though they were not forced to go to Carville by law, the stigma of the disease typically gave them no other choice. Julia Elwood came to Carville in 1956. In a 1999 Discovery Channel documentary, *Banished: Living with Leprosy*, she spoke of her admittance to Carville: "It was very hard for me to deal with it. I kept praying and crying. . . . I thought I was coming to Carville to die."

In a 1976 interview, Elwood said, "I was only fifteen years old when this happened, so it was quite traumatic. I was afraid of it. One of the things about Mexican culture is that we are very religious. I had the biggest hell and damnation fear of it" (Bermudez B-8). Julia Rivera (Elwood) changed her name to Juliette Rivers at Carville. After she was released as a patient, she went back to Texas and earned a degree in education. Later she returned to Carville, serving as a public relations director and principal of the school. She was the first former patient to be hired as a member of the hospital staff.

Jose Ramirez Jr., now a social worker in Houston, wrote about the trauma he experienced during his diagnosis and admittance:

> The first time I was referred to by the "L" word was on the day of my diagnosis in 1969.[4] After months of going to physicians, dermatologists and *curanderos* (folk healers), I was finally diagnosed with Hansen's disease, more commonly known as leprosy. The public health official who informed me of my diagnosis attempted to reassure me that there was "nothing to fear" and that I would soon be back on my feet. He was telling me this while referring to me by the "L" word. My family was morbidly silent and the hospital initiated a strict plan of isolation, forcing visitors and medical staff to be shrouded in caps, gloves, and masks when entering my room. (Ramirez 2002: 2)

Ramirez says that he was transported from his hometown of Laredo, Texas, to Carville in a hearse, allegedly because there were no ambulances available (Ramirez 2). He entered Carville on February 22, 1968, later attended Louisiana State University, and received a degree in social work.

In the personal narratives of former Carville residents relating the circumstances and events of learning that they had leprosy and that they would be "banished" to Carville for isolation and ineffective treatment, there are many of the characteristics of trauma and trauma narratives. The narrators remember feeling total devastation. They also experienced a feeling of impotence or total loss of control over their own lives and identities. They would be taken away from their families, homes, and the lives they knew and sent to live out their days in the hospital at Carville, usually under an assumed name. Their feelings of helplessness and fear were also accompanied by a need to remain silent about their trauma away from Carville.

As Cathy Caruth says, trauma has come to mean "a wound inflicted not upon the body but upon the mind" (1996: 3), and certainly it was the idea of being a "leper" that was often most traumatic for the victims. Caruth further says, "trauma is not locatable in the simple violent or original event in an individual's past, but rather in the way that its unassimilated nature—the way it was precisely *not known* in the first instance—returns to haunt the survivor later on" (1996: 4, italics in original). While it is unlikely that the trauma of a leprosy diagnosis was *immediately* assimilated by the patient, there does not seem to be the element of continuing unassimilated trauma and belated recognition. Caruth's theory of trauma as "unclaimed experience" does not seem to apply, as a whole, to HD patients.

For HD patients, the trauma "haunts" them from the very beginning. There is not the phenomenon of lost and recovered memory, often the case with violent, acute trauma. The memory of the trauma for HD patients is not repressed, though it was often silenced outside of the Carville community. The trauma and devastation of the experience seems to have been always there for elderly HD patients. Typically if they left Carville, it became a silent memory because they could not talk openly in most cases. It became silent memory shared only with "insiders," family members or friends who knew. For Carville patients, the initial shock or trauma became a kind of chronic traumatic state. As one patient said, "You never forget you have this disease." It is not something left behind but becomes part of one's continuing identity.

Caruth also argues "that trauma is not simply an effect of destruction but also, and fundamentally, an enigma of survival" (1996: 58). She says that one must recognize this paradox between destructiveness and survival to be able to recognize "the legacy of incomprehensibility at the heart of catastrophic experience" (58).[5] Caruth poses the question, "What does it mean to survive?" (60). Again, Caruth's theories do not wholly apply. While the enigma of survival as an escape from a real or feared threat of death is a part of most trauma narratives, the irony for leprosy patients is that historically they had to survive the threat of being considered the *"living* dead." Hansen's disease, in itself, is not fatal. The real fear before effective treatment and cure was ostracism and survival in a disfigured body. They were daily reminded by bodily signs that they had not escaped. The violence and destruction were coming from within their own bodies.

Most studies and theories of trauma narratives are based on traumatic experience that involved violence against the person and often physical wounding by another person or group—for instance, holocaust narratives and child sexual abuse narratives (see, for example, Caruth, Culbertson, Brison, Kaufman, Ramadanovic, et al.). These involve a dimension of human evil perpetrated by another human being—a willful violation of another person's body or personal space or rights for the benefit of the violators. In these trauma narratives of evil violation, silence is a factor, and eventually putting the experience into narrative form can be a therapeutic act or survival strategy. However, there is *never* a time when the victims can look back on the traumatic event with a sense of playful humor, though perhaps with ironic or black humor. It certainly never becomes a source of humor or entertainment for others.

In the Carville narratives, the diagnosis, the separation from family, and the forced confinement to

Carville, Louisiana—often for a lifetime of ineffective treatment—were indeed traumatic for the victims. The narratives reflect the same horror, loss of identity, and need for silence. They differ, however, in that the narrators are eventually able to see the trauma as a result of human *ignorance* and *fear*, not deliberate human evil. There is also a realization that they suffered from their own ignorance as well as that of society, its quarantine laws, and its response to a bacterial disease.

Eventually, these "victims" of trauma are able to establish a life in Carville or elsewhere, to reconstruct their identity. They have survived what seemed insurmountable, and they have often found personal happiness within the new community or on the "outside" when they left Carville. Most important, they can laugh at society and often at themselves for responding as they did. Of course, some do respond with anger and hatred for the system. More commonly, however, they are able to come to some understanding of their treatment as uninformed or as informed by fear. While the disease may be regarded as "evil," they do not attribute evil to the people whose decisions led to their ostracism. They understand the folly of human fear and ignorance. They also have lived to see the triumph of medical science over the leprosy bacterium, at least in the United States and countries where medical treatment is widely available. Their traumatic experience is part of a narrative of triumph against the evil of a bacterial disease.[6]

It is significant for the study of trauma, memory, and narrative that the traumatic memories of the diagnosis and entry to Carville do not seem to have been repressed and later recovered. Even for those who later silenced their memories on the outside, there was a time at Carville where they could openly talk about their own experiences and memories with those whom they knew had undergone similar experiences. Every patient at Carville had shared a similar trauma and had the advantages of community. This, of course, did not justify the legal quarantine. Carville was always a very real prison for those confined there, but the community that the patients created could also serve as a safe haven. For those who remained at Carville, there was always a potential community in which they could speak about the trauma and share experiences and stories. As misguided as isolation and a kind of quasi-quarantine with several weeks of official leave per year may have been, the Carville community of patients provided an in-house residential support group where stories could be shared. Perhaps the greatest determinant of the dynamics of trauma, memory, and narrative is the powerful effect of a community of people who shared the same experience. This effect is evident not only on the kinds of narratives constructed but on the processing of traumatic experience, memory, and survival.

The effects of community, the lack of violence and deliberate human evil in the traumatic event, and the fact that recognition of the trauma could not be postponed for those who were forced to enter Carville all contribute to the responses of the patients. In general, patients came to a realization that they could rebuild their lives and reconstruct their identities.[7] Part of this process was weaving their experiences into narratives of their own. Gussow and Tracy wrote in their 1968 study of Carville patients, "They formulate a theory of their own to account for their predicament, to de-discredit themselves, to challenge the norms that disadvantage them and supplant these with others that provide a base for reducing or removing self-stigma and other-stigma" (319).

The narratives of traumatic experience and memory were not, of course, recorded at the time of crisis but later—to therapists, journalists, folklorists, anthropologists, and to each other. They worked through the trauma and the need for silence to tell their own stories and to provide a counternarrative to the prevailing cultural narrative about leprosy. Hilde Lindeman Nelson uses the term *counterstory* for a story that resists an oppressive identity and attempts to replace it with one that commands respect. She says that counterstories are "tools designed to repair the damage inflicted on identities by abusive power systems" and that they "resist, to varying degree, the stories that identify certain groups of people as targets for ill treatment" (2001: xiii). She further says, "The counterstory positions itself against a number of *master narratives*: the stories found lying about in our culture that serve as summaries of socially shared understandings" (2001: 6). Counterstories seek to alter the dominant group's assumptions as well as the "oppressed person's perception of *herself*" (7), serving as "narrative acts of insubordination" (8, italics in original).

I prefer to use the term *counternarrative* in regard to the Carville personal narratives. It helps to avoid the suggestion that *counterstory* may sometimes imply that these are fictionalized accounts and moves the texts farther from the implications of *tale*—overtly fictional narratives. Counternarrative is a more neutral term, and it also seems more comprehensive as a description of the body of personal narratives from Carville. While counternarratives in general play against the dominant or master narrative of a culture, the counternarratives from Carville seem to engage and challenge not only a master narrative but two separate (though related) master ideologies. They are playing against both an ideology of morality based in the Bible and the ideology of a legal system that said they could not live in society, use public transportation, or exercise their rights as citizens (for example, the right to vote). The Carville patients created a sort of ideological neutral space where they could construct their own narratives to counter the effects of the biblical narrative (especially Leviticus) that they were morally "unclean" and the effects of the legal narrative that they were physically "unclean" and thus a threat to society. They were trying to find a way to live in a culture whose ideological system and master narrative said, "You do not get to live." Their counternarratives provide a text of their refusal to accept the dominant narrative and system of ideas.

From almost the very beginning, there were counternarratives from Carville. Certainly the narratives were first of all a way of dealing with trauma and reconstructing their own identities and sense of self. Early stories perhaps show most poignantly their pain—that they were people, not *lepers*, who were being exiled to Carville. Later stories were used, in the words of Stanley Stein, "to radiate the light of truth on Hansen's disease" and to promote the rights of the patients. The stories told in the 1980s and 1990s continued to have a political agenda, particularly those that gave details of being forced to come to Carville. They were used, in part, to pressure the federal government to maintain the HD Center at Carville.[8] Most important, Carville patients told stories to make sense of their lives—to deal with the past by giving it a structure in narrative and to create the possibility of a future for themselves. In the words of folklorist W. F. H. Nicolaisen, "We tell stories because, in order to cope with the present and to face the future, we have to create the past, both as time and space, through narrating it" (1993: 61).

{ 3 } "Through the Hole in the Fence"

PERSONAL NARRATIVES OF ABSCONDING FROM CARVILLE

The patient has to start by treating his illness not as a disaster, an occasion for depression or panic, but as a narrative, a story. Stories are antibodies against illness and pain.

—ANATOLE BROYARD
Intoxicated by My Illness

Illness is not all tragedy. . . . Much of it is funny.

—ANATOLE BROYARD
Intoxicated by My Illness

Because there are so many misconceptions about leprosy patients, the sense of isolation continued for many of the older patients in the 1980s and 1990s, even though they were all there by choice. The continuing use of the term *leper* to denote an outcast from society was particularly evident during the late 1980s in comparisons of AIDS patients to "lepers." This insensitivity, even among scholars, continues. Writing in 1995, Julia Epstein says: "In another time, those who are HIV-positive would be wearing the leper's bell, the Jew's yellow star, or the homosexual's pink triangle as symbols of outsiderhood and its attendant and contagious depravity" (167). Because of the sense of being apart from others, the older patients at Carville continued to tell personal experience stories and other tales about their lives and how they dealt with the horror and fear associated since biblical times with the words *leprosy* and *leper* and with being forced to live their lives separated from the rest of the world.[1]

Among the most fascinating stories told by the older residents of the Hansen's Disease Center were the tales about leaving Carville illegally during the time when leprosy patients were confined to Carville by law. Until the 1940s there was no effective treatment for the disease, and a diagnosis of leprosy was virtually a lifetime sentence to Carville. It was not a real quarantine since patients were permitted short periods of official leave after an initial time of treatment, usually to visit their families. However, they were prohibited from using public transportation and they were compelled by law to return to Carville at the end of the official leave. There was no federal regulation for compulsory treatment or isolation at Carville, and the laws of individual states differed. In addition, the state regulations for quarantine of HD patients were repealed at various times from 1950 to 1976, so there is no date that marks the end of compulsory isolation.

There seems to have been a unique sense of community among the patients at Carville, particularly before the 1960s, when there was still compulsory or strongly urged isolation. Yet, their common bond was that they were victims of a disease and were not there by choice. Because they could not accept a life of imprisonment for having a disease, many patients left the hospital illegally, "through the hole in the fence." Some were discovered on the "outside," arrested, and returned to Carville. Many, however, chose to return voluntarily, facing a sentence in the Carville jail for absconding, because the trauma of being fugitives and the fear of being discovered as escaped "lepers" were worse than the prospect of spending the rest of their lives in a leprosarium.

For many, absconding was a very uncharacteristic thing to do, and the decision to go through the hole in the fence was traumatic for them. For others, mostly men or young men, it was a kind of game or recreation to try to beat the authorities. No one took too seriously the absconding for a few hours or even a few days, and this was seldom even reported, but to leave for an extended time without access to treatment was considered serious.

In 1983, when I began studying the folklore, customs, and holiday traditions at Carville, I talked with people who had been at Carville when there was still compulsory isolation. Several people told me about their own personal experiences of absconding (Carville's official term) and then returning. These narratives provide a study of traditional beliefs about leprosy and the effects of the stigma from the perspective of the patient. They also make a statement about society that is perhaps even more important than the personal factor. Though they are personal stories told by people who had departed illegally, they differ in some respects from other types of escape narratives, such as prison escape narratives, slave narratives, border-crossing stories, and stories of AWOL (Absent WithOut Leave) soldiers.

In talking about life at Carville before the 1940s, Louis Boudreaux, an editor of *The Star* (Carville's official publication), said, "In those days, when we came here, we were here for life, most of us. And—most people who left here in those days went through the hole in the fence, and not the gate" (Personal interview 1983).[2]

I had first noticed the term "through the hole in the fence" to describe a common means of leaving Carville in Betty Martin's *Miracle at Carville*. She says that she and her fiancé, Harry Martin, a patient she had met at Carville, lost faith in the effectiveness of the treatments and the probability of a medical discharge. She also knew that with proper precautions, they would not be a threat to anyone on the "outside." They had, in fact, been out on passes and visits. She says:

> At first, when we had learned that many patients left Carville, singly or in groups, "through the hole in the fence," which is Carville lingo for absconding without discharge, we had thought it very wrong. But we had seen that most of the patients discharged were old or prematurely old burnt-out cases,[3] with little or no vision left, or so badly crippled that they had no person left to take them in, so they stayed on, broken and old, to end their days in Carville. . . . Discharge in those days was meaningless. It came too late. (Martin 1950: 90)

Betty and Harry Martin knew that health authorities and sheriffs would be alerted if they left. Since they had not given their true identities or addresses, there was little chance of their being found. They left at night, after cutting a hole in the barbed wire fence, and their fathers were waiting in a car behind the levee. They returned voluntarily six years later because Harry Martin's case had become worse, and he needed the institutional care that was the only care available then, however inadequate.[4]

In his autobiography, *Alone No Longer* (1963), Stanley Stein also talks about absconding. Though Stein never left Carville for an extended time, he says that he and a friend went "through the notorious hole in the fence" to go to fish fries on the levee and to get whiskey from bootleggers. He also helped others to escape, though he says, "Escaped lepers were deemed dangerous" (59). Stein says that Jimmy Houdini, a patient, "was given the name of the great escape artist because of his legendary departures through the hole in the fence. On one occasion . . . he took a whole group of patient friends with him" and "they all lit out for Texas." They were discovered when they rented a house and threw a party that continued an entire weekend (105). It was not the escape that was legendary but what happened later. Stein also says that often if a wife or husband was discharged, the other spouse would go through the hole in the fence.

In a 1975 article in *The Star*, Ray Elwood, a former patient who came back to Carville to work and later served as editor of *The Star*, talked about his episodes with absconding when he was a patient ("Man in Demand" 8–10). He came to Carville as a teenager in the early 1950s, when there was effective treatment. Often, however, he and his friends went through the hole in the fence, particularly on weekends in search of "unofficial" recreation. In the article, Ray tells the story about how one time they were discovered on the "outside." In an interview in 1986, he told me the following version of this particular episode:

This happened about 1950, about thirty-five years ago. We were a bunch of teenagers here, and one of the guys had a car, and he kept it behind the levee. We'd put our money together to buy the gas, and every weekend, we'd leave and go to New Orleans or Baton Rouge, and this one weekend, we were out late in Baton Rouge and we decided to stop and get some coffee before we went back. So we went to the bus station, and a patrol car pulled up and the detectives started asking us questions—what we were doing out that late. I stayed sort of back—I was sitting on the curb. But this one guy couldn't keep his mouth shut, and he told them we were Merchant Marines from New Orleans and of course, we didn't have any papers, so he told them something else. So, one of the policemen radioed for a backup and the other one started frisking us. Then the two backups arrived, and they told them, "Every one of these guys has a different story." I was still sitting on the curb and one of the back-ups looked over and said, "Ray, is that you?" Then he said, "Ah, I know these guys—we played ball with them in the River League. They're okay—they're from the leprosy hospital." The detective who had been frisking us jumped back five feet and started rubbing his hands on his clothes. The detective who knew us started laughing and put his arms around us and said, "Don't worry—they're safe." (Personal interview 1986)

This version is basically the same as the printed version.

Rita,[5] another "absconder," was seventy-eight years old when I interviewed her in 1983. She first came to Carville when she was twenty, and after seven years, she married another patient who was twelve years older than she. They could not get married in Carville, so they left to get married when they were on a pass. They returned to Carville for a while and then left through the hole in the fence. She said:

> I went through the hole in the fence with my husband. We went to Hot Springs, Arkansas. I'll never forget that. We lived there a year. We knew a doctor there who had been here. And we went to visit him. And he was a good doctor. But when we went there, he played a dirty, dirty, dirty, dirty trick on us. He got the Board of Health there to send us back. And then you know what they did? They put us in prison [in Arkansas]— not in anything else—in prison. Dirty! No sheets or toilet, mosquitoes, mosquitoes, oh my God. And he used to come to visit us, and I'd turn my head, and I wouldn't talk to him.
>
> He did that to us! And I told him, "I don't want to speak to you—and don't forget—I thought you were a son of a Christian, but you are not Christian. I wouldn't talk to him—I'd turn my back every time he came.

And we stayed in there nine days before one of the
doctors from here came to get us in an ambulance—a
station wagon ambulance. And I had a blue dress on. It
looked like dirt—it looked like dirt when I left there.

And they had some sailors in there. My husband had
some cigarettes, and uh, so, and one of them passed by
and he said, "Y'all the ones here that got the leprosy?"
He said, "Y'all ain't got that. Y'all look too good for
that." He thought it was traditional in the old, old days
when they used to say about that, you know, that your
fingers would fall off and everything. Man—did I laugh.
We had us an experience. (Personal interview 1983)

Hazel, a native of St. Louis, was eighty-five years old
when I talked with her in 1984. She had been a discharged patient since 1946, but she came back to
Carville in 1969 because of cataracts. She said that
when she first came to Carville in 1922, "Once you
came in—you couldn't go out that gate. I thought I was
here and that was it. But things changed over the years."
She said:

I ran away one time—went through the hole in the
fence. Them days we just had a barbed wire fence. All
kind of holes in it. I left in '46. A colored man, we called
Preacher—he came with his little Ford—and I went
through the hole in the fence. And oh, I had wrote my
father I was coming. . . . I wouldn't go back to St. Louis
because I was running away and I was scared because

anytime you run away, they notify the authorities where you come from they look for you—so I went to Chicago. . . . [Her mother and father met her and they lived there six years.] And one time we were in Chicago, going down Madison Street, and we were at a fruit stand, and I saw a couple coming down the street, and I said, "Oh, my God, Mama, don't look at them." I was afraid they would recognize me. It was my best girl-friend, and I ignored them. If I had talked to her, she would have gone back to St. Louis and told everybody, and they would have come looking for me. I came back on my own free will. And then, when you came back if you didn't have someone to go your bond for you, you went to jail. A man I knew in Carville went my bond.

I got tired. I wanted to go home, and the only way I could leave was through the hole in the fence. . . . I went home with two suitcases and a steamer trunk. Some of the young men helped carry them to the car. (Personal interview 1984)

She laughed as she ended the story, and she said that most of the people there, at that time, did at one time or another go through the hole in the fence. Hazel died at Carville in 1985.

Mary Ruth was eighty-two when I first talked with her. Both Mary Ruth and her husband, Darryl, came to Carville in 1939, when Mary was twenty-two. She said of her husband, "He was my first love, and I married him. He was going to run away, in 1941, I think, and join the service. But he had a reaction and he couldn't leave." Darryl died in 1998, and Mary Ruth still referred to him as "my Honey" until her death in March 2004.

When I asked Mary Ruth in 2001 if she had ever gone through the hole in the fence, she said:

> Oh, yes. Definitely. And I enjoyed it [laughter]. We
> used to go see LSU play football. Every Saturday
> they played at home. And when LSU was playing in
> Mississippi. We went to Alabama too. But we didn't go
> through the hole that time—we got a pass. We had to
> go by car and all that. We had a Corvair. The times we
> went through the hole, we had no way to go out, and
> we had to rent a car. And a bunch of us got together
> and paid twenty-five dollars. And twenty-five dollars
> was a lot of money at that time. We had eight of us.
> We had to squeeze in. (Personal interview 2001)

Mary said that a friend or relative from the outside would rent a car and come to pick them up. They would hide to leave, and Mary hid in the trunk of the car. Once they went through the hole in the fence to go to an LSU game, and when they got to their seats in Tiger Stadium, they realized that one of the doctors from Carville was sitting a few rows in front of them. "Oh, yes. And Nippy Carville and her husband were with them, and Dr. Erickson was there. He never looked back, but Nippy did. So at halftime, we changed seats. We went up higher [laughter]. Oh, I loved Nippy. And she called me, and said, 'Where'd y'all go?'" Nippy

Carville was the mother of political analyst James Carville.[6] She died in early 2001. The town of Carville was named for the Carville family. Mary said that later another doctor saw the car, but that was the only time anyone saw them in the stadium: "Of course, they all knew we were going through the hole, but they kept it under the hat. They didn't call us down. Only one time they called, and said, 'Just be careful.' Because people see the car. We weren't married yet. That was in the 1940s. We had to look for tickets when we got there." Mary said that later, in 1960, they got season tickets. "So every year we'd get tickets—charge them on our Visa cards. By the 1970s, we didn't have to go through the hole. . . . Well, I was the only one who was in the trunk [of the car]—inside the trunk." When asked if they had to go through the hole in the fence to get married, Mary Ruth said:

> Oh, no, no. We had a pass. But at that time, Louisiana people got only ten days [official leave] and Texas people got fifteen days. But I went to the doctor and I told him—Dr. Jo—[Dr. Johansen], he was my pal. I said, "Dr. Jo, we going to get married." And he said, "Well, let me know if—" but you had to pass the blood work. And my Honey had it all figured out, what he was gonna say. And he was drinking, but the blood was all right. But one of the other patients' blood was bad— they saw something, and it wasn't syphilis that they

had seen, but they wouldn't marry them. So from that
experience, he said, "I've been drinking all night."
Last thing—they gave us a dinner party—I forget the
name of the restaurant.

Mary Ruth also told about going through the hole in the
fence for a trip to New Orleans after they were married:

We were having a drink—I think that's the only time I
had a drink [laughter]. We went through the fence to
go to nightclubs [pause]—at the Blue Room [a very
posh dance club in the former Roosevelt Hotel in New
Orleans]. Who ever thought that we'd see anybody over
there. So, we were having a drink, and this lady—I
didn't know her, but I found out afterwards who she
was—said, "How are you? How's everybody in Carville?"
I mean, *out loud*. Ah, Lord! All of us could have gone
through a hole, you know. And Vivian, you know, said
she was never going back to New Orleans after that.

Mary said that she found out later that the woman who
recognized them was the wife of the editor of the *Times-
Picayune*. She also said that she and her husband took
many vacations, "visited twenty-four or twenty-six
states." She said: "We went to the World's Fair in 1964.
There were eight of us in two cars. We had a lot of fun.
And we got lost one time, and we had said if we got lost,
we would meet at the stable in Maryland—Annapolis.
We'd meet there because [her brother] wanted to show

Mama Annapolis, because he was in the Navy. We went
to New York when the World's Fair was in New York."
Because she was a Texan and they were married, Darryl
also got the two weeks.

Though some Carville residents absconded without
literally going "through the hole in the fence," there
was in fact an actual "hole." In the Carville centennial
publication *Known Simply to the Rest of the World as
Carville* (1994), Julia Elwood gives the specific location
of the "hole in the fence":

> The infamous "hole in the fence" was located close
> to the end of the road by House 29. It was used before
> the 1960s when the administration would not permit
> passes for patients to go out to shop or for any other
> reason. Someone had dug out enough dirt for a person
> to fit under the fence and people could tell that there
> was a well traveled path through it. Many a patient
> would "abscond" through it to visit their families or
> to go take in a good high school or university football
> game. After an "absconded" patient would return, he
> would be placed in jail for from two weeks to 30 days
> for leaving "against medical advice." (1994: 42)

Johnny Harmon also gives a colorful description of
"the hole" in his autobiography *King of the Microbes*:

> In the south east corner of the eight foot hurricane wire
> fence was "THE HOLE." Next to the hole was the river
> road. I don't know who cut the hole but it was always

open. If you wanted to take a swim or fish in the Mighty
Mississippi River you went through the hole. If you
wanted to go out to a near by town there were ways
of getting in touch with some one to take you. A ren-
dezvous was arranged and they would pick you up at
the hole. The hole was approximately a quarter of a
mile from the front gate and around a slight curve. I am
sure the powers that be knew about the hole but this
was not Germany or a hostile country so no one ever
got shot going through the hole. (1996: 36)

Johnny Harmon met his wife, Anne Triche Harmon, at
Carville in 1936, and they were married in 1948. They
lived on the hospital grounds in a small cottage built by
Mr. Harmon. Their two children, a son and a daughter,
were born while they were at Carville. Because children who were free of the disease could not remain in
Carville, a couple from Vacherie, Anne's hometown,
cared for them. Johnny Harmon was released in 1954;
Anne Harmon remained at Carville until 1957. After
their son was born, Mr. Harmon writes: "We visited our
son every chance we got and the Becnels would come up
on weekends to see us. Anne and I would crawl through
the famous hole in the fence and we would have a picnic
under the willow trees on the back of the Mississippi
River" (88).

The feelings of the patients about absconding are certainly understandable. They had been permitted passes

for visits home, and no worker (medical or other) in the history of Carville has ever contracted the disease. Yet they were not permitted, until the 1960s, to leave the hospital voluntarily or to ride on any form of public transportation because they were considered menaces to public health.

Historically, the isolation of leprosy victims was not based on empirical or scientific data, but on irrational, fear-based attitudes that regarded leprosy as punishment for sins and a physical manifestation of a spiritual disease. Leprosy was not perceived as being contagious in the same way as most other contagious diseases—such as plague. Since most people exposed to leprosy did not contract the disease, the alternate explanation of punishment from God was generally accepted. Peter Richards discusses the history of the treatment of leprosy patients in his book, *The Medieval Leper*. He says: "The convention that lepers should be separated from society runs through eight centuries of European history. . . . The tradition that fear of infection was the common key to the isolation of lepers is oversimplification. No aspect of the leper's history is more important, because attitudes toward him were closely bound up with reasons for setting him apart" (Richards 1977: 48). Saul Nathaniel Brody says in *The Disease of the Soul: Leprosy in Medieval Literature* that there was in medieval times a "striking disparity between the stringency of laws enacted to contain lepers and the laxness with which they were enforced" (1974: 91). He further says, "the laws were unenforceable or at least unenforced." Brody points out that "the leper's physical suffering is compounded by the anguish of his exclusion from the world. He fears isolation as much as he fears death" (1974: 91). This dichotomy of stringency of laws and laxness of enforcement was still very much a part of the management of leprosy in the early part of the twentieth century, and this is evident in the narratives about absconding from Carville. By the twentieth century, the knowledge that leprosy was a bacterial disease and was, in fact, contagious reinforced earlier fears in the United States and led to quarantine laws by states. The enforcement of the law was not as clear once a patient entered Carville. "Absconders" could be pursued by local authorities in their hometowns if their whereabouts and identities were known, while at the same time other residents were given passes for a week or more for home visits. This may be why authorities at Carville, though certainly aware of holes in the fence, may appear to be lax in eventually looking the other way while residents absconded.

Dealing with the *stigma* of the disease (along with the necessity for secrecy) is always a part of narratives about absconding from Carville. Because of the stigma attached to the words *leper* and *leprosy*, patients in

general use the term HD to refer to the disease. In talking about the stigma in the historical context, they may
use the word *leprosy*, but they were not likely to use
any of those terms openly in the past. Even today 95
percent of leprosy patients do not tell anyone their diagnosis, except for close family members; they are usually treated at outpatient Hansen's disease clinics or by
private physicians.

In writing about personal experience stories, Sandra
Dolby Stahl says, "the story teller's own values influence the perception of experience, encourage the casting
of the incident in a story form and prompt the repetition
of the story in various contexts" (1983: 270). This seems
to be true for the personal experience stories about
absconding told by Carville residents. How the tellers
perceived these incidences was obviously influenced by
their own knowledge of the disease and the misunder-
standings that resulted from the lack of knowledge and
understanding on the part of "outsiders" and the incon-
sistencies of the laws and regulations.

That these stories and the attitudes and values
expressed in the stories are typical not only of these
patients but of Hansen's disease patients in general
seems evident from the number of such stories that are
told and from the fact that the personal narratives, in
some cases, are repeated by others or, in other cases, are
reported in print. Though personal narratives may be

performed only for the interviewer (see Clements 1980: 106–12), this is clearly not the case with these narratives. They were well known in the Carville community, and they seem to express the strong personal attitudes of Hansen's disease patients toward their treatment by "outsiders" and by the law. Dolby Stahl has contended, "The personal narrative is the most likely vehicle for expressing a traditional attitude since it represents an incident, an actualized behavior pattern" (1977: 21; see also Labov and Waletzky 1967; Bauman 1972; Langellier 1989). These stories encode what came to be a traditional pattern and attitude among patients, but they also express the very personal attitudes of the absconders. They not only report but justify a behavior that occurred quite regularly because of this attitude. In this sense, there is a traditional core of content in the absconding stories, and this differs from typical personal narratives. In addition to providing entertainment and humor, the absconding stories function as statements about the relationship of the "escapees" to society and how they dealt with it. They also reflect society's values and make judgments about them. They make a powerful statement about a society that ostracized its members (regarded them as social "lepers") because of a disease (actual "lepers" in the society's terms).

The structure of the personal narratives of absconding seems to reflect both a need to provide a frame of reference for the audience to understand the actions of the teller and a need to show that rather than being defeated, the teller triumphs in the end. Each story usually begins with a justification for absconding. Then there is a statement about the "escape." This involves no personal risk or danger and if any details are given, they are usually humorous. Next there are the actual details of the experience of being on the "outside," whether the stay was very brief or extended. Finally the teller relates either the reason the decision was made to return voluntarily or, if forced to return, a humorous incident that results from the situation, usually from the reactions of the "outsiders." In either case, the teller shows that he maintained some control over the situation. The humor in these stories seems to function in somewhat the same way as the humor in any tale where the underdog triumphs. They tend to poke fun at the stupidity and prejudices of "outsiders" as viewed by the folk community at Carville. There is also the violation of boundaries, not only physical ones. The absconding stories, in the way they deal with boundary crossing with impunity, seem analogous in function to the Brer Rabbit tales for slaves and ex-slaves and to other trickster tales. As John Robinson has pointed out, recounting an achievement or triumph over adversity reaffirms "man's ability to control his affairs." Robinson also discusses the importance of the ludic

motive in personal narrative (1981: 60–64). This motive
seems especially important in the absconding stories.

Obviously, the absconding stories originally depended
on the esoteric factor (see Jansen 1959). These stories
were told almost exclusively to the "in-group." The narrators had little contact with others, the absconding stories tell of things clearly against the law at that time, and
the function of control and humor would be only a part
of an in-group audience's reaction. The "in-group," however, would include not only those who had the disease
but also those who "understood." The "outsiders," those
at whose expense the stories are told, are those who had
no understanding or accurate knowledge of the illness
and who were, in fact, believers in the common misconceptions and stigma of "leprosy." The patients and former patients could openly talk about their experiences
for publication. It is quite possible, however, that there
was a more intimate sharing of stories only among the
former residents that would still not be shared with any
other person.

In this respect, the absconding narratives are much
like other personal escape narratives. As with the leprosy
patients, there was a clearly defined "in-group" audience
for narratives of former slaves, prisoners, AWOL soldiers,
or border crossers. Like the Carville patients, they too
often included details of events after the escape, "close
calls" of being discovered and humorous details of how

they outwitted authorities or outsiders. There are, however, major differences between other types of escape narratives and the Carville narratives.

In the other personal escape narratives, the story usually focuses upon the escape itself, or at least the escape is a crucial part of the narrative that relates a plan with some danger and the process of overcoming the danger and outwitting authorities. This is not the case in the Carville stories. The escape was easy and done routinely. Carville authorities knew it occurred regularly, and they made little effort to deal effectively with it. For the young men, such as Ray Elwood and his friends, the regular "escapes" were adventures, with no real peril at all. In addition, the Carville patients were regularly given passes to leave, as long as they had clearance to travel through any states on their routes home. There was no armed guard to hold them in, and patients usually had at least one month of leave per year. In this respect, when they absconded they were somewhat like AWOL soldiers in that the escape itself was usually not perilous. They were merely absent without leave. For prisoners, there had to be an escape plot, which was at least an attempt to be different from others, and there was always grave danger. Prison narratives tell of such things as guards shooting a prisoner trying to escape, without any warning or chance to turn back. Bruce Jackson points out that stories about legendary escapes are part of every prison's folklore (1972 and 1965). The same is true of other types of narratives that involve escape. Robert B. Klymasz says, "A true border-crossing story points to the obstacles that test and that, of course, try one's mettle and purity of intentions" (1983: 229). In describing the slave narratives, Arna Bontemps says they always began with a description of the "Negro's suffering in his private hell of oppression." He endured this until he "eventually was impelled to attempt the perils of escape." His expectations were "A promised land and a chance to make a new life as a free man" (1969: vii). For those who went "through the hole in the fence," there were no perils of escape, and there was no real hope of a promised land.

In all the narratives, the absconders returned voluntarily or remained in Carville voluntarily after they were no longer required to be there. Narratives by escaped prisoners, draft dodgers, illegal aliens, and ex-slaves do not typically relate a voluntary return—though escaped prisoners perhaps acted in such a way as to insure their return (see Jackson 1978). However, stories of AWOL soldiers do show that they often turned themselves in before the time had passed for the AWOL charge to be automatically upgraded to the more serious charge of "desertion."

Finally, the absconding narratives differ from other escape narratives in that the leprosy patient was most likely to be "turned in" by those whom he mistakenly thought he could trust. Unlike the slave whose skin color made him a suspect to everyone, the person who absconded from Carville could seldom be identified by any signs of the disease. The former slave, however, could rely on his friends, sympathizers, and the Underground Railroad to help him. For leprosy patients, so much depended upon who knew the real nature of their whereabouts and diagnosis. If they had not given their real names or hometowns upon entrance, they perhaps had only to fear the doctor who had diagnosed the disease. As Philip Kalisch points out, there was little compassion for an "escaped leper" (1973: 525).

Considering the intensity of the stigma attached to leprosy, it seems likely that it was this stigma more than anything else that led Carville patients to escape and subsequently also led them to return. As Goffman points out, for the stigmatized individual, the stigma becomes the pivotal factor or focus for identity by others and for self-identity (1963: 5). For Carville patients the stigma had usually come upon them suddenly, with little warning, and through no fault of their own. Nothing in their lives could have prepared them for it—unless they had a relative who also suffered from the disease. Most typically, however, they were likely to share the popular beliefs about leprosy.

Though certainly the desire for freedom and the desire to have options in one's life functioned as motivations to abscond from Carville, just as important was the need to escape from the psychological trauma of suddenly being hit with the ultimate stigma and at the same time losing one's former identity. Most who decided to return after a long absence say that they returned because they got tired of "hiding" and because they needed medical treatment. Equally important is the probability that they could not escape the stigma of leprosy. Psychological escape and social acceptance were probably the greatest needs, but the stigma was so deeply embedded that this was seldom possible. For many it was easier to deal with in Carville.

Clearly, the older residents of Carville continued to tell these stories about absconding because the telling of the stories was rewarding to them and created a sense of intimacy. Julia Elwood heard these stories as a former patient who returned to Carville as a staff member. She said: "Old timers get together, and they really come up with some humdingers. They enjoy getting together and telling these stories" (Personal interview 1986). In a highly esoteric group of patients or former patients, entertainment and intimacy, a bonding together of "those who know," seem the primary motivations. The intimate feelings are known and shared. When the absconding stories are told to others, however, the motivations seem to be different. While they seem to be sharing the details of the experience, some painful but many humorous, they seem to be establishing a kind of bond with the listener to let him know that they had faced the adversity and overcome it. More important, however, is the fact that these stories do not blur the reality (for the narrators or the listener) of the inhumane treatment by society. They show quite clearly how society reacts to leprosy. It is not that they all overcame the stigma, but they were perhaps saying that they have given up on dealing with a stigma that was almost impossible to overcome; instead, they laughed at the society that imposes such a stigma.

The absconding stories have basic similarities to and differences from personal narratives, escape narratives, and possibly tales dealing with psychological or socio-cultural boundary crossing. If these stories continue to be retold and particularly if they are repeated by the children and grandchildren of former patients, it seems likely that they would eventually become legend material. While they do not fit neatly into any one established genre of folk narrative, one hesitates to ascribe a special genre designation to the absconding stories because of the very limited focus. It would be interesting, however, to compare narratives from other leprosy hospitals in Hawaii and other countries or even from other types of hospitals to the Carville narratives.

The stories of outwitting the authorities or frightening those on the "outside" gave Carville patients a common bond, and also provided a kind of control over their lives in a situation where much control had been lost. The absconding narratives, playing with both the esoteric-exoteric difference in attitudes toward leprosy and the violation of the quarantine, provided and continue to provide for them a way of defining their relationship with society and coming to terms with a society that rejected them. These personal experience narratives continue to help them to maintain their identity as persons and to maintain a feeling of having managed, in the worst of circumstances, to retain some modicum of control over their lives. They show the patients wrestling with the need to escape but finding the boundaries they most needed to cross basically sociocultural and psychological, not physical. They could not overcome the stigma, but they can laugh at violating the boundaries set by the outside world.

{ 4 } Telling It Slant

PERSONAL NARRATIVES, TALL TALES, AND THE REALITY OF LEPROSY

Tell all the truth but tell it slant—
Success in Circuit lies
Too bright for our infirm Delight
The Truth's superb surprise.

—EMILY DICKINSON

Humankind cannot bear very much reality.

—T. S. ELIOT
Murder in the Cathedral

For most people, the truth's "superb surprise" of having someone say to them "I have leprosy" is more reality than they can accept or even fathom. Some people may not even be aware that Hansen's disease still exists in the United States or that there is even a possibility that former leprosy patients might be sitting next to them. In fact, it is so unreal to most people that references to leprosy are almost always regarded as a joke. The possibility that someone is telling the truth when saying, "I have leprosy," seems to be frightening and threatening to people whose only associations with leprosy may be from the Bible and *Ben Hur*. Images of the hooded person carrying a bell and shouting "Unclean, unclean" when anyone approaches quickly come to mind. Because of this, people who have this disease learn that it is much more adaptive to "slant" the truth in dealing with the realities of leprosy.

In an article on leprosy and stigma, Philip Kalisch notes: "About 95 percent of the patients outside Carville leprosarium concealed the nature of their illness from all but very close family and friends since they knew from their own and others' experience that they would not be hired by a prospective employer if it was known that they had or did have leprosy" (1973: 531, note 125). Kalisch further says: "There has almost always been a deep primitive fear of leprosy in men—a fear often times reinforced and overladen by religious fear. . . . But unlike other social stigmas of mankind (racial, for example) Americans did not think leprophobia incompatible with Christianity. On the contrary, such a view, in loyal union with the supreme code of Leviticus, only strengthened the incarceration movement. It made possible the cleansing from society of an evil force" (1973: 524–25). While some former patients, like Johnny Harmon, did speak openly about their illness, in general, most patients and former patients could only hope that their "secret" was not discovered. In a 1975 article in *The Star*, Julia Elwood describes the trauma experienced not only by herself and her husband but by her children as well as a result of "rumors" in the neighborhood that they had leprosy. She says: "What happens when this piece of news gets to the persons who delight in spreading garbage? Besides the fact that damaging news travels with ultra-sonic speed, it invariably hurts innocent bystanders. Take, for instance, children of patients. They go to school along with the rest, at the same level, but only until that fateful day when someone utters in a miasmic whisper, 'My parents say I can't go to your house because your daddy has leprosy'" (1975: 6). She then asks the question, "Are these children outcasts? Why?" (6).

Hansen's disease is a real illness, but leprosy is a term that historically has maintained metaphorical meanings inspired by medieval beliefs, which cause emotional responses far out of proportion to any threat or danger. In *Illness as Metaphor*, Susan Sontag discusses how a disease, such as leprosy, takes on metaphorical meaning, particularly if it was historically an incurable disease whose cause was unclear. She says:

> First, the subjects of deepest dread (corruption, decay, pollution, anomie, weakness) are identified with the disease. The disease itself becomes a metaphor. Then in the name of the disease (that is, using it as a metaphor) that horror is imposed on other things. The disease becomes adjectival. Something is said to be disease-like, meaning that it is disgusting or ugly. In French, a moldering stone façade is still *lepreuse*. . . . Feelings about evil are projected onto a disease. And the disease (so enriched with meanings) is projected onto the world. (1978: 58)

Speaking of the context of disgust in the high Middle Ages, William Ian Miller says, "Lepers were the most polluting of beings; unlike Jews, who could pass unless identified with special badges and apparel, they disgusted on sight. Even high rank did not save the leper. . . . they were banned from all company except that of other lepers" (1997: 154).

Though the intensity of the leprosy stigma in the United States may have diminished by the late twentieth century, the stigma still exists despite the fact that patients are of no danger to society. For example, a 1987 *New York Times* article was headlined: "Uproar Over

Plan to Treat Lepers." The piece begins, "Fear and resentment swept over Alviso, Calif. when residents learned of a plan to treat 176 leprosy patients at a community clinic." It goes on to say, "The Family Health Foundation which operates the health center decided against treating lepers primarily because of the public's reaction" (Oct. 18, 1987, p. 65). *New York Times* reporters, at least in 1987, were apparently not aware that being referred to as *lepers* is particularly odious to HD patients and in fact is regarded as the equivalent of a racial or ethnic slur.

Sontag suggests that the disease metaphor is made obsolete by an understanding of cause and a cure. Evidence suggests that this has not really happened with leprosy. Perhaps one of the reasons for the continued dread of leprosy is the long time between discovery of the cause and discovery of a cure or effective treatment. In addition, the general public was never really aware of a treatment, as such. There is more of an assumption that the disease had "disappeared," at least other than in Third World countries. The disease may have "disappeared," but the metaphor stayed. Sontag says in *AIDS and Its Metaphors*: "Even the disease most fraught with meaning can become just an illness. It has happened with leprosy, though some ten million people in the world, easy to ignore since almost all live in Africa and the Indian subcontinent, have what is now called, as part of its wholesome dedramatization, Hansen's disease, after the Norwegian physician who, over a century ago, discovered the bacillus" (1989: 93). In the popular mind, leprosy is not "just an illness." In fact, it seems to be perceived as not an illness at all, as far as most of the Western world is concerned. Rather, it is used almost exclusively as a metaphor, detached from any connection to a "real" illness (that is, an illness that one might actually get).

References to leprosy in the media and in popular culture are often not to the actual disease itself, though it is becoming somewhat more common because of comparisons to AIDS and because of the extensive media coverage that the closing of the Gillis W. Long Hansen's Disease Center in 1999 brought to Carville. It is also true that Mother Theresa and Princess Diana brought attention to the needs of leprosy patients, but these patients were almost always perceived as a "problem" of Third World countries. Instead popular references to leprosy are most often metaphorical. Sometimes it is a metaphorical reference to the ultimate horror of the past. For example, CBS News in 1988 said of Ivan Boesky, after he had received a three-year sentence for illegal trading on Wall Street, "He has become a leper in the business community." Referring to children with AIDS, Dr. Matilde Krim, president of the American Foundation for AIDS Research in New York, said,

"These children are truly the new lepers" (*U.S. News and World Report*, July 7, 1986, p. 7). More recently, Al Hunt, on CNN's *The Capital Gang*, referred to someone as "an ethical leper" (Aug. 24, 2002).

Most often, however, contemporary references to leprosy are humorous metaphors. In the movie *Grease*, a girl says, "I have so many hickies, people think I'm a leper." In *Good Morning, Viet Nam*, Robin Williams's character says, "If someone in America says 'Slip me some skin,' they're not a leper . . ." A booklet in a mail order catalog is entitled "Do Diapers Give You Leprosy?" Humorous references to leprosy are made on television shows. On *Kate and Allie*, when the children are sent upstairs, one of them asks, "What are we, lepers?" On *Golden Girls*, Blanche, posing as a nun, tells a priest, after he has overheard her conversation with a man: "He's a leper. I'm the only one who'll touch him." Rex Reed, in a review of the horror movie *Corrupt*, compares the appeal of the movie to that of a "a convention of lepers." In *Lake Wobegon Days*, Garrison Keillor has Father Emil, the Catholic priest, tell Sister Arvonne his thoughts on why he objects to the blessing of the animals on the lawn of Our Lady of Perpetual Responsibility on the Feast Day of St. Francis. He says, "I think, Sister, we could bless animals without having them on the premises, same as the criminals or lepers—you wouldn't ship in a bunch of lepers so we could pray over them, would you?" (1985: 190). This, of course, was written to be humorous, to evoke laughter. Keillor earlier mentions that his family made him feel like a "leper" (1985: 110).

The effect on HD patients of hearing the word "leper" used as a metaphor is illustrated by a 1938 entry by Sister Hilary Ross in her Carville journal:

> Over a year ago the 1937 World's Series was played, and whether you were for the Giants or the Yankees, you know it was a thrilling series—thrilling even if listened to over the radio. And the patients down in Carville listened to it . . .
>
> Well, the day of one of the games every patient was listening to the broadcast, forgetting for the moment their oft-times multiplied pains of body and mind. Now just at the close of the game the genial and jocular voice of the announcer said: "Well, the umpire, you know, the umpire is the Leper of the game. Everybody despises him but nobody touches him." Oh, the pity of it! Could you have seen the joy drain from their faces and the hard bitter looks as the radios were switched off. (Qtd. in Elwood 1994: 46)

The intensity of the leprosy stigma and at the same time the "unrealness" of the stigma as something that could, in fact, actually befall a person is illustrated in the only two references to leprosy by Erving Goffman in his book *Stigma: Notes on the Management of Spoiled*

Identity. In dealing with information management and whether or not to try to hide a stigma, he says: "medical officials who discover a case of leprosy may suggest that the new secret be kept among the doctors, the patient, and his immediate family, perhaps offering this discretion in order to ensure continued cooperation from the patient." (1963: 95). Later in the book Goffman says that in dealing with a stigma, "In addition to matter-of-factness, levity is also recommended." As an illustration of the successful use of humor in dealing with a stigma, he quotes Macgregor, et al.: "A somewhat sophiscated female patient whose face had been scarred by a beauty treatment felt it effective upon entering a room of people to say facetiously, 'Please excuse the case of leprosy'" (1963: 116, quoting Macgregor 85). Goffman quotes this without comment, and in effect, simply does not address how a real Hansen's disease patient would deal with the stigma. He does show, however inadvertently, the double view of leprosy in popular culture as both the ultimate stigma and as humorous metaphor.

Because of the stigma caused by popular beliefs about leprosy, patients with Hansen's disease have learned that it is best to slant the truth—if the truth must be dealt with at all. Many former Carville patients tell stories about their own experiences in dealing with what to say to outsiders. These personal narratives show both the traditional attitudes of the community toward outsiders and the personal experience of the teller with outsiders.

For many older patients there was never again a successful "normal" relationship with society after they came to Carville. In the past, many former patients have established normal relationships with society by keeping their illness secret. Ray and Julia Elwood, who came to Carville after there was effective treatment, have lived relatively normal lives on the "outside" but continued to work at Carville until their retirement, when they moved to Texas. They have become "spokesmen" (to use Goffman's term) for Hansen's disease and work to eradicate the stigma through education of society. Julia tells, however, of how she and her family were affected when the "news" of their illness reached unsympathetic ears.

Most former patients who have established identities "outside" do not tell these stories except to very trusted, close family members or when they come back to Carville for medicine or visits. Betty Martin tells her story in *Miracle at Carville* and through many interviews in the ten years before her death, but she never revealed her real name.

It seems that these stories, at least at one time, were told only to insiders and trusted friends. Ray Elwood, a former patient who later became editor of Carville's international publication on Hansen's disease, *The Star*, agreed that these stories were usually told within the community and that some of them could not have been told openly. He gave the following example:

> When we were teenagers, almost every week-end we'd go into New Orleans or Baton Rouge. We went to movies, football games, dances—and many of us had girlfriends in Baton Rouge or New Orleans. The girls never knew—we told them we were from St. Gabriel [a town near Carville] and we didn't have a phone. We told them we would go to a neighbor's house to call them for a date. We would never have told anybody about these things then—we especially wouldn't have wanted the parents of the girls to know—every parent in Baton Rouge and New Orleans would have wondered if the person their daughter had dated was one of us. We were the lucky ones—we looked like any other teenagers. [There was effective treatment then.] (Personal interview, Feb. 1986)

For Ray Elwood and other patients who are treated before there were any outward signs of the disease, the question of dealing with the truth may involve only covering one's tracks about where one has been or what one is being treated for. Older patients who have deformities resulting from injuries caused by the loss of sensation (anesthesia caused by nerve damage) or from bone absorption must contend with questions about their condition. Usual responses are "I was in an accident," or "I was burned" or "War injury." One personal narrative, however, may be on its way to becoming a legend in the extended Carville community. I first heard this story from Julia Elwood about a patient who was known for his exploits and stories:

> He's a character—he can tell this story better than I can. He's got what we call mitten hands—all of his bones have absorbed, through wear and tear and carelessness and so on. So he has two hands that are kind of mitten hands. He has a thumb on both of them. And so here he is—and he's very versatile, a very spirited person, very active. He goes all over the place—he plays pool, he goes to drink beer at the canteen, goes to all the activities that we have, sings in the church choir, a very good person. He's just really active. He's around sixty-two or sixty-three years old. But, ah, he stayed out as long as he could, and he tells this story where he was in this night club and they asked him what was wrong with his hands, and he says, "I'm going to tell you two stories, and y'all choose which one you want to believe." So he says, "I was in Korea—in the battle zone—I went up the hill and there was bombs all over the place," and you know, he was setting the scene of this war, like, and he says, "Me and my buddies were in this jungle and this bomb exploded, and both of my hands were mutilated— and they had to operate and everything. And, the other story is I have leprosy." And everyone went, "Ha, ha, ha, ha, ha. Of course, you were in the war." It just breaks

> me up every time he tells that story. And he says,
> "Everybody thinks I was in the war. I gave them a
> choice." (Personal interview, Jan. 1984)

This tale not only illustrates a tradition of telling these
stories but also suggests the reaction of at least one
in-group person to the performance of the narrative and
the role of the original performer. Julia Elwood is not
simply retelling the story. She is telling about the original narrator's telling of the story. Though the original
narrator was clearly identified as someone known to
the person repeating it, this story seems on its way to
becoming legendary.

I later met with Billy, the original narrator, and he
told me the story. Billy first came to Carville in 1952.
His doctors discovered a problem when he was about fifteen, in about 1938. They thought it was polio. According to Billy, he went to the Mayo Clinic in 1946 and was
diagnosed as having a nerve disorder. In 1952, he came
to Carville, after being diagnosed by a doctor in Florida
who had been at Carville. Though there was treatment
then, he already had extensive nerve anesthesia and
limb damage. He was at Carville from 1952 to 1957,
when he was given a medical discharge. When he left
Carville, he worked with heavy equipment and in construction in Florida and Louisiana and on the construction of Interstate 10. That is how his hands continued to

be injured. In 1952, there was still compulsory isolation at Carville, but there were vacations and passes to leave. Billy also left many times illegally, "through the hole in the fence."

Billy was away from Carville for over twenty years. He came back voluntarily in 1976, not because of the Hansen's disease but because of other health problems. He worked in the laundry and continued to drive his car and, in general, to be fairly self-reliant. In March 1986, I met Billy at Carville, and he told me several stories, including the story about fooling the sailors in a bar. I had been visiting Carville for over two years at that time and had heard about Billy, but he had never been there when I visited (usually around holidays or semester break, times when he was usually away, traveling or visiting friends). This was the only time I spoke with Billy. He died later that year.

Billy was outgoing and friendly. When I asked him about the story in the bar, he laughed and said: "Nobody can deny I wasn't in Korea." I asked, "Were you in Korea?" He said, "I've never been out of the United States. Nobody can deny I *wasn't* in Korea." Then he proceeded to tell me the story:

> I was in this bar—it was a nice bar. When I go into one, I usually try to find a seat by myself. Now, not that I'm anti-social, but, ah, I've never been the first one to

talk to someone, but if someone wants to talk, I go along with the conversation.

There was two seats on one side and three seats on the other, and I had my cigarettes in my hand and my drink on the table—and five sailors walked in, and two sat on one side and three on the other. And one of them was a chief petty officer, an old-timer in the Navy.

So, ah, I lit my cigarette, had my drink, you know. So, they watched me—saw how I smoked my cigarette, held my drink with two hands, and everything. And one of them asked me, said, "How you hurt your hands?" So I said, "Oh, you wouldn't believe it if I told you." And, ah, they said, "You were in an accident?" "You got 'em burned off?"

So I said, "I tell you what. You want to find out. I'm going to tell you the two stories. One of them is going to be the truth, and one of them is going to be a lie. I'm going to tell you the lie first. Then I'll tell you the truth after." I proceed to describe the territory in Korea where I was at—"I was in the Fifth Infantry, 405th Division"— They didn't know the difference; I didn't know the difference. "I was in the Korean foothills . . ." I described the territory— "Up there, about 500 foot or so—there was a little hill—we were supposed to take that hill at 0548. I had four of my buddies with me. We was going up the hill. We hit a foxhole, and they started opening up on us. I saw a Korean throw a grenade, and I reached up and grabbed hold of it—and I was going to throw it back, and," I said, "the thing exploded in my hands. The only thing that protected me was my helmet and my jacket. And my buddies saw them, and killed all three of them. And then my buddies grabbed my hands—wrapped my hands in a tourniquet—and they were going to take me to the first-aid station—about an hour and a half down the trail. But I said, No, I'd go by myself. So I was walking there when a sniper started shooting at me, and he hit me in the leg. I jumped off to the side, and he finally stopped shooting, and I started crawling. I didn't know I was crawling around in a mine pit—and all of a sudden, things started exploding and I was going through the air, and I didn't know what was happening. When I come to, I lay there five or ten minutes, trying to get my senses back and get my hearing back. I knew my leg was hurt, 'cause I had pain down there, and I started to get up, and it buckled on me. I looked down, and there was my foot—all mangled up. So I finally crawled to the first aid station, and they sent me back to the states, and that's how I got my hands and leg like that."

I said, "Now that's the lie. The true story is I got leprosy."

Everything quiet. Then [Billy goes into mock hysterical laughter, imitating the listeners], "Ha, ha, ha, ha, ha, ha."

One said, "You hear that. You hear what he say, man."

"Yea, I heard it."

"You believe that story—Ha, ha, ha."

"Let me see that hand."

"Yeah, that's a war injury."

It didn't cost me a penny the rest of the night.
(Personal interview 1986)

Billy said he first told the story about Korea after he was released from Carville in 1957. He was working in Civil Service for the Navy. He also told the construction companies he worked for that he had had a bone infection or the Korea story. He said: "I devised this story. I was on the bus from Jacksonville to here. I had my crutches, my foot was off, and some of my fingers. An elderly man on the bus asked me what happened to my hands. I said, 'You wouldn't believe me if I told you.' He said, 'You don't want to talk about it.' I decided to tell him what happened—told the Korea story. He believed it" (Personal interview 1986). Until his death in 1986, Billy performed this personal experience story/tall tale regularly. He also told me that this kind of experience had happened many times to him and that whenever he gave people a choice, they never "chose" to believe the leprosy story.

Billy also told a story on himself and the one time when he did not get away with attributing his injuries to Korea:

> The other day, I was going to Gonzalez [a town near Carville] on 30 and the police had a roadblock. The lady said, "May I see your license?"
>
> I said, "Pardon me, but I'm going to have to get out so I can get my billfold." So I went over to the side and got out and I was scratching like that trying to get my bill-fold out of my pocket. And so there was a policeman,

and he said, "Ah, forget it," and I said, "No, you want to see a driver's license, I'm going to get my driver's license."

So I got my billfold out. He said, "What the hell happened to your hands, man?"

I said, "Oh, Korea, hand grenade."

He said, "Oh, yea?"

So right there on my license it says, "U.S. Public Health Hospital, Carville, LA." So he says, "You at the hospital?"

I said, "Yea."

He said, "No problem."

(Personal interview 1986)

Billy was relating a personal experience narrative about having told a tall tale and being believed. He obviously enjoyed reconstructing the episode in the bar. Why did he tell the leprosy part? It was certainly not a need to tell the truth (evident from his story to the policeman) but clearly to dupe the "outsiders," not only by fooling them (he could have just said "war injury") but by fooling them with impunity since he had also told the truth. This would not have worked if he had only told the truth; they probably would not have believed him but may have been horrified if he said seriously that he had HD. They could have thought he was being hostile because he felt offended by their inquiries. He could have said it jokingly, as in Goffman's example, but then he would have been using leprosy as a humorous metaphor in the very way "outsiders" use it, which would further stigmatize leprosy patients.

Billy was an accomplished storyteller, telling a story about telling a story.[1] He did not use the episode with the old man on the bus as part of his repertoire. Fooling an old man—or worse, lying to him—could have shown Billy in a bad light, even though he made up the story to avoid offending the old man. Clearly, it is "putting one over" on a group of macho Navy men in a bar and then being included in their socializing that Billy wanted to relate.

The success of Billy's story, both in the bar and as a personal narrative retold later, depended primarily on three things. First, Billy's story in the bar depends upon the almost universal use of the word *leprosy* in our culture as both ultimate horror and as humorous metaphor. Secondly, there is the "exploitation" of the expectations of the typical tall tale. Finally, Billy's own personality and ability as a storyteller made the story successful both with the original audience and with the audience that later hears it as a personal narrative about having told a "lie."

When Billy told his story in the bar or elsewhere to outsiders, he was fairly certain that no one would believe he had leprosy. While leprosy is still regarded as a stigma, the reality of leprosy in the present is not something with which most people have any experience. It is, rather, the meaning attached to the disease, the metaphorical use of the term, that people react to. S. I. Hayakawa gives *leprosy* as an example of "words with built in judgments," which "communicate *simultaneously* a fact and a judgment on the fact" (1972: 68). He says we use terms such as "Hansen's disease" rather than "leprosy" to "avoid arousing traditional prejudices." He further says, "Because the old names are 'loaded,' they dictate traditional patterns of behavior toward those to whom they are applied" (1972: 69).

The metaphorical meaning of *leper* as an outcast or one excluded from society is usually included in dictionaries and is certainly the meaning that is most often used, whether as a serious comparison or as humor. Susan Sontag says in *Illness as Metaphor*, "The people who have the real disease are also hardly helped by hearing their disease's name constantly being dropped as the epitome of evil" (1978: 85). It is no easier for them to hear their disease's name used as a joke. In addition, scholars and writers who would not use racial or ethnic slurs tend to use the word *leper* as though it were not an offensive word that might cause pain to actual people.

When Billy says in the story, "I have leprosy," his listeners are set up to react to it as a humorous metaphor.

Since Billy does not fit the stereotype of an "outcast," they assume it is defensive humor and not something that could possibly be true. In addition, because of the way Billy presented and built up the Korea story, when he finally tells the truth, it is perceived as the "lie" typical of the climax of a tall tale. Billy's injuries, however, must have some explanation, and the alternative to Billy's actual "lie" is so unacceptable that the listeners accept it (that is, the actual "lie") as true or, at least for the time, pretend that they do.

In *Story, Performance, and Event*, Richard Bauman says that "tall tales start out as apparently true narratives of personal experience, offered to be believed, with their ultimate effect traditionally derived by gradually bending the account out of shape—stretching the bounds of credibility bit by bit—until it finally reveals itself as a lie" (1986: 103). In a later article, Bauman says: "The special quality of the tall tale resides in its interactional effect, in the way in which the audience's response is exploited by the genre. The tall tale is manipulative in distinctive ways. . . . They aim to elicit the kind of belief accorded to personal experience narratives. . . . At some point in their telling, tall tales begin to challenge the belief of the hearer as they transcend the bounds of credibility and shift into the hyperbole central to the genre" (1987: 210–11). Bauman points out that tall tales challenge the sense of reality for the hearers, and "their reactions of astonishment and unfamiliarity serve as devices to help induce the tall tale response pattern, the shift from the 'this is true' of the personal experience-like opening of the tall tale to the 'is this true?' of its transitional phase" (1987: 215). The typical tall tale continues, "ultimately carrying the account to a level where it can no longer be believed" (1987: 218).

Billy's story is not a traditional tall tale, but the audience is set up to react to it as though it were. What is perceived as the "hyperbole central to the drama" of the tall tale (by the listeners in the bar) is actually a shift to the *truth*. At the end of his story, Billy uses the term *leprosy* literally (an actual disease), and this is what transcends credibility for the listeners. Therefore, they must interpret it metaphorically, with two options. Note that there is not an immediate reaction, but a pause ("Everything quiet") before the reaction. Since Billy does not conform to the metaphorical image of an outcast, they interpret it as a humorous metaphor or joke and accept the first story (the "lie") as true. We cannot be sure, of course, whether the men in the bar really believed the Korea story. It is possible that they did not. In a typical tall tale, the listeners finally see the entire story as the "lie" it is but respond with humor. Even if the listeners in the bar actually did discern the truth, Billy's story had diffused "reality" to the extent that they did not have to deal with it.

As Bauman points out, tall tales challenge the sense of reality and lead the listeners to evaluate the ambiguities of appearance and reality (1987: 215–17). Billy's narrative also deals with appearance and reality. Billy is relating a personal narrative about telling a *fabrication*[2] (he calls it a "lie") and also telling the truth in the bar. Though not a typical tall tale, his narrative in the bar builds up to a climax and follows the course of a typical tall tale. Thus, the audience's reaction is manipulated in the same way as the traditional tall tale. Like a tall tale, it challenges their sense of appearance and reality. This obviously would not have worked in the bar if Billy had told the truth first.

In Billy's tall tale, *he* is in control. He has knowledge the others do not have, also typical of tall tales. Billy is also consciously manipulating the in-group audience's reaction, and his personal narrative has evolved into a rather sophisticated use of metanarration. In telling about the experience in the bar, Billy moves in and out of the "bar" narrative with expertise, clearly aware of how he is framing the story and commenting on it. There are no previous recordings of this story, but Billy had recognition within his own community as a good storyteller. His narrative seems like a text that has been told many times and probably has expanded in length and use of metanarration over the years. He sets up the metanarrational frame very carefully, creating an illusion of reality but also making clear that it is an illusion (see Babcock 1977: 70) by commenting on the narrative. (For example, "I proceed to describe the territory in Korea where I was at—'I was in the Fifth Infantry, 405th Division'—They didn't know the difference; I didn't know the difference.") It is notable that midway through the "Korea" part Billy stops commenting on the narrative, and the frame recedes into the background. The effect is that the later audience is also somewhat "taken in" by the tall tale.[3]

It seems that a recurrent theme in the personal narrative is the narrative about one's experience as a storyteller. Texas storyteller Ed Bell, for example, tells about having told a tall tale in "The Spotted Pup Award." Bauman points out that the Spotted Pup story is "essentially a metanarrational story about the telling of a story" and "it actually oscillates between the two" (Bauman 1987: 217–18). Billy's story is much like Ed Bell's story in that it recounts a fabrication and oscillates between the two. In addition, Billy seems to fit somewhat into the Münchausen tradition (see Dorson 1982: 77–174 and Ives 1988: 24–27) when stories about his storytelling are told by others. As Ives points out, "individual stories in the Münchausen's cycle are reports, not of events but narrations of yarns the Münchausen is said to have *told* rather than of deeds he is said to have *done*" (26).

It is interesting to compare the versions of the story given by Julia Elwood and Billy. Both include, "I gave them a choice," but in Billy's narration he also tells them which is the lie and which is true. In addition, Billy identifies the men in the bar as sailors, describes the bar, and in general includes much detail. Billy's matter-of-fact manner of presentation—in contrast to the content—is also typical of tall tales.

Also important is how Julia Elwood portrays Billy and how Billy portrays himself in the tale. In the case of Billy's story, one cannot make assumptions about what he is saying and why without considering also Billy's personality and the context of his repertoire of stories. Sandra Stahl has suggested the importance in personal narrative interpretation of "the link between the content of the narrative and the personality of the storyteller" (1988: 391). Billy's personality is described by Julia Elwood: a character, very spirited, very active, a very good person. Billy portrays himself in framing his story. He establishes early that he goes to a "nice bar" and that he is approached by the others—he does not go up to them. Billy then gives them two explanations for his injuries without technically deceiving them, and he is accepted socially. The closing is especially important: he becomes part of the group and they buy him drinks. The personal experience that Billy relates to his later in-group audience is the telling of a "lie" or story to a group of sailors, having them believe it, and becoming a part of the group for a night of socializing in a bar. He is accepted not only as "normal" but as somewhat "heroic" (or at least a very good storyteller). This is important to Billy—witness his closing line: "It didn't cost me a penny the rest of the night."

Billy's in-group audience certainly had a special appreciation for his particular situation in the bar and seems to greatly admire how he handles it. What appealed to the in-group listener is that Billy was using a common device of HD patients (slanting the truth—or lying) in order to avoid ostracism or at least an uncomfortable situation. He seemed not only to succeed but to be included in the socializing of the group. There are, of course, two stories being told. In the first, the one told in the bar, we do not really know exactly what the men believed; we only have Billy's story for how they reacted. Of more importance is Billy's later personal narrative about his experience as storyteller. The in-group audience enjoys Billy's personal narrative about telling a "tall tale" because it is a situation with which they can clearly identify. If they have physical deformities, they are likely to have been put in the uncomfortable position of explaining them without mentioning leprosy or Hansen's disease (which people may know is "really" leprosy). If the situation is a transient one, there is usually no real problem, but few HD patients have not had some experience with being ostracized when their illness was discovered. These experiences range from a passenger getting up and taking another seat on a bus, to a child's birthday party being boycotted because the word had somehow gotten around the neighborhood that the parent had been treated for HD, to denial of employment.

Erving Goffman calls "taking off" on (joking about) fooling "normals" a "sad pleasure" (1963: 134). Goffman says: "The person who very occasionally passes often recounts the incident to his fellows as evidence of the foolishness of the normals and the fact that all their arguments about his differentness from them are chuckled over, gloated over by the passer and his friends" (1963: 135). It seems to me that calling this a "sad pleasure" is inaccurate in the case of leprosy patients and especially with Billy. Billy routinely hid the real cause of his deformities from others. While he may have chuckled over his "lie," it seemed important to Billy not to offend other people, and he obviously enjoyed socializing. Though he did indeed seem to deceive the "inquirers" in the bar, he certainly did not cause them any harm (though *they* might think differently, if they knew). The real pleasure came not from Billy's ability to "pass" but from the telling of the story.

Because of Billy's storytelling ability, he managed to avoid an awkward situation and, at the same time, do what HD patients know they cannot do—that is, tell the truth. It is likely that many people would have difficulty with someone next to them (on a plane, in a bar, and so forth) saying, "I have leprosy," not because of any danger to themselves but because people do tend to respond to meaning-laden terms with traditional patterns of behavior. Billy's storytelling ability enabled him to subvert the stigma and gain social acceptance without sacrificing any of his personal integrity. When he shaped and retold his experience in the bar, he was glorying in his performance as a storyteller, and also humorously reinforcing the point that the reality of leprosy and the images it conjures up are so far apart that people will accept this story even when he told them he was lying to them, and said, "The truth is I have leprosy."

{ 5 } The World Downside Up

MARDI GRAS AT CARVILLE

With masks, when visitors came, they had nothing to fear.

—SISTER HILARY ROSS

In the world of carnival, the awareness of the people's immortality is combined with the realization that established authority and truth are relative.

—MIKHAIL BAKHTIN

Michel Foucault begins the first chapter of *Madness and Civilization* (1988) with this statement: "At the end of the Middle Ages, leprosy disappeared from the Western world." He goes on to say,

> Leprosy withdrew, leaving derelict these low places and these rites which were intended, not to suppress it, but

to keep it at a sacred distance, to fix it in an inverse exaltation. What doubtless remained longer than leprosy, and would persist when the lazar houses had been empty for years, were the values and images attached to the figure of the leper as well as the meaning of his exclusion, the social importance of that insistent and fearful figure which was not driven off without first being inscribed within a sacred circle. (Foucault 1988: 6)

As Foucault points out, leprosy was widespread in medieval Europe.[1] "Lepers" were regarded as "witnesses of evil," and "in a strange reversibility that is the opposite of good works and prayer, they are saved by the hand that is not stretched out" (1988: 7). Foucault argues that during the Renaissance, insanity and mental illness replaced leprosy as a moral scapegoat. He says, "Leprosy disappeared, the leper vanished, or almost, from memory; these structures remained" (1988: 7).

While Foucault may be correct in his argument that the insane, like those with leprosy, became stigmatized by their illness, he is inaccurate in his assertion that leprosy disappeared with the Middle Ages or that the image of leprosy vanished from memory. Though leprosy was no longer endemic in Europe, it certainly continued to exist. Indeed, the medieval images of leprosy are still alive today. In 1995, Mississippi novelist Barry Hannah wrote:

I had heard throughout my life the curious rumor of a leper "colony" down in south Louisiana. *Colony*

> evoked folks lost in an exotic fastness. . . . *Leper* of
> course was as bad as it got, poor devils. . . . At Carville,
> where I finally got over forty years of mildly curious
> ignorance, I saw the doubloons from last year's Mardi
> Gras at Carville were imprinted on one side with an
> armadillo. On the other was the Federalist infirmary
> building: *Gillis W. Long Hansen's Disease Center 1921.*
> (Hannah 1995: 40, emphasis in original)

The juxtaposition of Foucault's ideas of "inverse exulta-
tion" and "strange reversibility" regarding leprosy with
the symbolic inversions of carnival, and more particularly, of Mardi Gras at Carville, may evoke a weird sense
of the carnivalesque. The carnivalesque world upside-
down is challenged, decentered, reversed upon itself
when the carnival inversion includes those who historically have been the ultimate Others.[2] Mardi Gras at
Carville provided participants with a creative context
whose potentialities for symbolic inversion and meaning through ritual performance were quite different
from those of other carnival participants.

Mardi Gras in New Orleans and other areas of south
Louisiana is an important calendar festival that cele-
brates the last day before Lent. The exact structure of
the festival ranges from the street parades and elaborate
society productions of carnival balls in New Orleans
and other urban areas to the true folk festivals of rural
southwest Louisiana's *courir de Mardi Gras*. Mardi

Gras for the Krewe of Carville followed the general structure of urban Mardi Gras celebrations in Louisiana, with costumes and masks, a parade with music, food and drink, favors or tokens being thrown or begged for, general revelry, role reversal, and symbolic inversion.[3] It was unique, however, in that the participants were residents or staff members of the Gillis W. Long Hansen's Disease Center in Carville. More important, the symbolic inversions of carnival and the function of transformation from masking and performance had special dimensions for revelers who lived with the stigma of leprosy.

An unusual and subtle effect of transformation occurred in this ritual at Carville. To act in a carnivalesque mode is to be allowed the freedom to be "abnormal" for a while. Paradoxically, to celebrate Mardi Gras, like other masquerade holidays, is normative—it is not only allowable but even expected that one will participate in the seasonal customs, particularly in Louisiana. Thus, for people who are already stigmatized as "abnormal" in society, the masks and the occasion allow an opportunity to engage in normative behavior, to act "normal." In the carnival world of make-believe, the residents at Carville could perceive themselves as "normal." It was a reversal of the typical festival inversion. The reversals at Carville were often not from taking on "deviant" roles; rather, people who were stigmatized and regarded as "deviant" took on "normal" (in terms of Mardi Gras) roles or even exalted roles. It was another inversion of the carnivalesque "world upside down," with subtle dimensions of appearance and reality.

Mardi Gras at Carville very early took on the tone and the characteristics of carnival in New Orleans, perhaps because of the presence of patients from New Orleans who wanted to continue to observe their traditional Mardi Gras celebrations. Betty Martin writes in *Miracle at Carville* that her father described Mardi Gras as "the time when the whole population of New Orleans, plus visitors from all over the country, turned out en masse to escape reality" (1950: 10). She says that she "loved the novelty of being someone else for a day, the fun of watching thousands of maskers in beautiful or comic costumes parading on the avenue between the throngs of people" (1950: 10). The year Betty Parker Martin was nineteen (1927) was particularly important to her because she had been recently engaged to a medical student in New Orleans. Between Christmas and Mardi Gras that year, she was diagnosed with leprosy, was compelled to leave New Orleans, and went to Carville for treatment. In 1931, she went to a Mardi Gras dance and masquerade at Carville with Harry Martin, the patient whom she later married. She writes, "Mardi Gras was being held in New Orleans. I thought of St. Charles Street and the parades

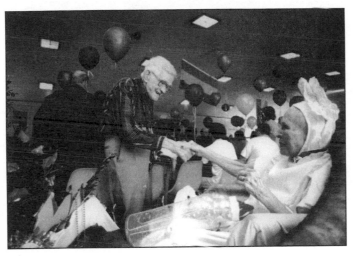

*Johnny Harmon and Betty Martin, Mardi Gras at Carville,
1998. Photo by Jeffrey Braverman.*

and costumes that are part of our heritage of make
believe dear to my childhood, dear to every New
Orleanian's heart. . . . Here in Carville we, too, held carnival . . . and the crowd in costume might have been any
crowd in New Orleans" (Martin 1950: 79). Betty Martin,
whose appearance was unmarked by the disease, continued to participate in Carville's Mardi Gras. In 1995, she
dressed as a cancan dancer, with a red and black costume
complete with ruffles, fringe, and mask. In 1996, she was
Cleopatra, with a costume and a wig of long, straight

black hair, reminiscent of Elizabeth Taylor's portrayal in the movie. In 1998, she was dressed as a baby doll in a carriage.

Louis Boudreaux, former editor of Carville's official publication, *The Star*, had many memories of Mardi Gras at Carville. When I spoke with Boudreaux in 1984, shortly before Mardi Gras, he had been at Carville for forty-nine years. Both he and his late wife, Kitty, had participated in Mardi Gras. Speaking of the early Mardi Gras at Carville, he said:

> Then, there was compulsory isolation. . . . Then, there was considerably more togetherness. You weren't going anywhere, so you had to make the best of a bad situation. I think that's why celebrations in those days were quite different than they are today. A person coming in today is thinking of getting out as soon as possible. . . . The ones that maintain the celebrations are the ones who have been here a long time. Mardi Gras was one of the big traditional celebrations here. We had beautiful miniature floats, the parade, and of course, a beautiful ball. We elected a king and queen. In the old days, it was up to the various patient organizations to put this on . . . and they worked real hard at it. There was the Lions Club, American Legion Auxiliary, Patients Federation, and the American Legion Post here . . . and one of the oldest organizations here, the Latin American Patients Organization, had a club, called the Mexican Social Club, and it still exists, and they also had a float. And

the Music Club had a float. So you see, we had so many
local organizations. It was more like a community
than a hospital. (Personal interview 1984)

Although concealing identity was no longer as much of
a priority for older residents in the 1980s and 1990s,
it was clearly important earlier when patients were
encouraged to change their names when they entered
Carville to protect their families. Louis Boudreaux had
stressed how important it was to conceal his identity
when he entered Carville in the mid-1930s. Concealing
identity with a mask, however, is part of Mardi Gras
fun, not to hide but to play.

Johnny Harmon also remembers Mardi Gras as an
especially important event at Carville. He spoke with
me in 1996 about the early Mardi Gras celebrations at
Carville:

> I came in '35, and the Mardi Gras came up in '36. . . .
> I dressed up like Mae West. We had a big time. In those
> days, we were a world of our own. We couldn't go out
> the gate except for twice a year. We were isolated. And
> there were enough of us that we had a world right here.
> And believe it or not, time didn't drag either. When we
> were well enough, we got into everything. The sisters
> were so good about promoting things. They were won-
> derful. You know, outside of their regular jobs—Sister
> Laura was a music teacher—and they had some real

good musicals, Christmas plays and so on. And the Mardi Gras, we would start working on that a few months in advance. We'd build things—and some of the floats were real elaborate. I was the King one year [1937]. Kitty [wife of Louis Boudreaux] was Queen. (Personal interview 1996)

Johnny Harmon, of course, was one of the few former Carville patients who did not conceal his illness or his identity after he left Carville. In his autobiography, *King of the Microbes: The Autobiography of Johnny P. Harmon*, which was privately published in 1996, he gives a description of his first Mardi Gras at Carville:

The next big event to take part in was the patients' own Mardi Gras. I decided I would masquerade as Mae West. I wrote to my sister Myrtie in Texas and she helped me get the necessary paraphernalia together. My sister made the dress and bought me a wig and all the accessories I needed to get my act together. . . . We built our floats on anything with four wheels that was adaptable to the walks. Since I was a draftsman and had also studied commercial art, I got into the designing and building months before Mardi Gras day. When the day arrived we paraded the walks and wound up in the recreation center's ball room. After all the toasting and protocol was over, there would be a dance and all out celebration. Folks said I made a real convincing Mae West and I had a lot of fun playing the part. (Harmon 1996: 27)

In a later entry, Harmon compares Mardi Gras in 1994 with those in the past: "Feb. 18, 94, was Mardi Gras and the patients, as usual, had their Mardi Gras celebration. Bicycles, wheel chairs, and various carts were decorated and converted into floats and competed for prizes. . . . With the reduced patient population the patients' Mardi Gras are not nearly as elaborate as they were in 1937 when I was the King" (1996: 167). Johnny Harmon also includes photographs of himself and Anne Harmon as Carville Mardi Gras king and queen.

Billy also had many memories of Carville's Mardi Gras in the 1950s. Billy said that there were extraordinary floats in the parade, which was along the corridors (wide covered and screened walkways that connect the buildings). The dance was upstairs in the ballroom of the recreation building. In an interview with me in 1986, he said:

> They had dances. They had floats. It's much different now. Then it was a closed community, and people were here long then. . . . There even were some children, teenagers. Visitors could come in.
>
> We'd build our own floats . . . we had different themes. One float I remember was supposed to be a pirate ship. And there was a Hawaiian here. He made a wonderful, wonderful pirate. This one, I remember [laughter]. Of course, we had plenty of cats, just like we got now. And, all of a sudden, just before Mardi Gras, all the cats started disappearing. "What happened to the

cats? Where'd the cats go? Somebody must be shooting them." And so, the night of Mardi Gras, at the end of the ballroom, Billy Hall had a float. . . . On it, they had a great big treasure chest. And when they got to the ballroom—there were about 200 patients on one side and the Sisters [of Charity] of the other—they opened the treasure chest, and cats by the dozen come out! Running everywhere—one went under a Sister's robe. That was a sight to behold. Chaos! You'd have to be here to believe it.

It was different than it is now. It was a real community. Had a king and a queen. The patients would vote on the king and queen. Kept secret, and it was presented the night of the ball. (Personal interview 1986)

A photograph of the pirate float described by Billy from a Mardi Gras in the 1950s was published in Carville's centennial publication (Elwood 1994: 62).

These accounts of Mardi Gras at Carville over the years reveal fond memories of special times of celebration. Certainly, there was a sense of community among the residents, who considered Carville a world apart. While the residents were from diverse backgrounds, they took on the carnival spirit of role-playing and fantasy within their community. Like other carnival performances, there was also role reversal, transgression of boundaries, and chaotic play, along with transformation and hidden identity through masking. In addition

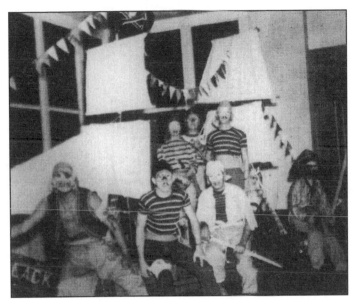

Pirate ship float, Mardi Gras at Carville, 1950s. Courtesy of National Hansen's Disease Program.

to the memories of residents, there are also published accounts from the print media, particularly from the Baton Rouge newspapers. Baton Rouge *State Times* reporter Ed Clinton published his observations regarding the 1957 Mardi Gras: "Carnival is a matter of spirit, of feeling. It can escape you even while you're standing in the midst of a half-million carousers as Rex, Lord of

Misrule, reigns supreme in the big one in New Orleans. Or it can completely captivate you as you stand in the covered corridors at this shut-away world at the U.S. Public Health Service Hospital here and watch the Krewe of Carvillians caper through their annual parade" (Clinton 1957: 1). The staff of the patient publication, *The Star*, provided insiders' views of the preparation and celebration of Mardi Gras at Carville through the years. Guided by *The Star*'s outspoken founder and editor, Stanley Stein, the publication recorded the triumphant successes of Mardi Gras celebrations, but it also took the opportunity to publicly admonish those who failed to honor their commitment to the patients at Carville. The 1957 article, "Mardi Gras at Carville Sparkles With Gaiety," is an example:

> Weeks of hard work went into preparations for the carnival with Louis Boudreaux, Patients Federation Entertainment Chairman, and Fred Smith, veteran carnival-ier, as the mainsprings. Everything went smoothly and beautifully except for one disappointment. A Baton Rouge orchestra sent here, courtesy of the Musicians Union Transcription Fund, arrived "too little and too late." The orchestra held up the parade for an hour or more and then dwindled from an expected seven pieces to three—the alibi: "we got lost on the way." They must have also lost their "music." The background music for the court ceremonies was anything but effective and

the sound they made for music was a conglomeration of
cacophony. But even this musical mishap did not let
down the high spirits of the carnival revelers for it was
truly the night in Carville that "Care forgot." (8)

Until the late 1980s, the Mardi Gras celebrations
included a parade along the center's four miles of covered walkways. Later the parade and festivities were
held in the large ballroom, accessible to all from the
covered walkways. The floats in the parade were motor-
ized wheelchairs, large tricycles, or bicycles that had
been elaborately decorated to match the participants'
costumes. Since some of the residents at Carville were
HD patients before the 1940s, when sulfone drug treatments were introduced by Dr. Guy Faget to arrest the
disease, they had varying degrees of disabilities and
deformities caused by nerve damage and loss of sensation. They chose to remain at Carville because of the
difficulties of readjusting to the "outside."

In the 1980s and 1990s, it was this group of older residents who seemed most involved in the Mardi Gras celebrations. For these people, in addition to the social
interaction and conviviality, the Mardi Gras celebration
seemed to provide the more important function of transformation. The masks provided anonymity and hid
disfigurements, and the choices of costumes seemed to
suggest both a desire to participate in what is currently

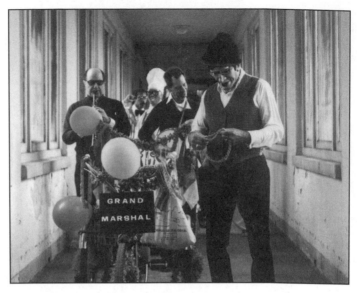

Mardi Gras wheelchair and bicycle parade, 1984.

popular in the outside world and also the carnivalesque inversions and play. For example, there were Pac-Man, J. R. Ewing, and E. T. costumes in the mid-1980s, as well as a Mike the Tiger, Louisiana State University's mascot. In 1989, there were Dolly Parton and Mike Tyson impersonators, a "Cajun Crawfish Boil" float, and a Surgeon General C. Everett Koop costume and float. Koop had visited Carville the year before, and his distinctive white beard and military uniform were parodied. Since all of the doctors and nurses at Carville are U.S. Medical Corps officers, who, like the surgeon general, dress officially in military uniforms (Carville was both a U.S. Marine base and a Public Health Service Hospital), military uniforms and personnel are often parodied. In fact, previous directors of the HD Center also held the position of assistant surgeon general of the United States. In 1995, then surgeon general Joycelyn Elders was parodied on a float.

In the 1994 Mardi Gras, shortly after the decision to end Carville's brief affiliation with the U.S. Bureau of Prisons, there was a float depicting the grave of the Bureau of Prisons with "B.O.P.—R.I.P" on the gravestone. The Public Health Service had signed an agreement in 1990 with the Bureau of Prisons to occupy half of the now 330-acre complex, which included offices, clinics, dormitories, homes, churches, a golf course, a lake, and streets lined with huge oak trees. Minimum-security federal prisoners lived at Carville and worked at certain jobs, such as serving food in the cafeteria. The official reason for terminating the agreement was the difficulty of maintaining adequate security at Carville. It is clear, however, that most HD residents did not like having prisoners there and were happy to see them go. The week before Mardi Gras, word of the planned float leaked out and caused quite a controversy. The Bureau of Prisons director wrote a letter of protest to the HD

Center director at the time, Dr. Robert Jacobson, demanding that the float not be allowed in the parade. Jacobson reportedly responded that the B.O.P. did not understand what Mardi Gras is all about and refused to intervene. The float was a great success, and the morning after the parade, a picture of the float appeared on the front page of the *Advocate*, the Baton Rouge daily newspaper—to the great delight of the Carville residents.

Adding to the general revelry and the spirit of the participants, Father Frank Coco and his Jazz Musicians provided music for the Carville Mardi Gras from the 1970s through the mid-1990s. Typically, the Jazz Musicians, led by Father Coco, were at the head of the parade, leading the revelers as they threw out beads and doubloons. Father Coco, a jazz clarinetist and a Jesuit priest for more than forty-five years, was a chaplain at Our Lady of the Oaks Retreat House in Grand Coteau, Louisiana. He was also a chaplain for Pete Fountain's Half-Fast Walking Club, which parades in New Orleans on Mardi Gras. Mardi Gras at Carville was usually celebrated on the Friday before Mardi Gras, enabling Father Coco as well as some Carville residents to go to New Orleans on Fat Tuesday. In addition, Mardi Gras day is a holiday in southern Louisiana, even for many federal employees, and only a minimal staff of doctors, nurses, and other essential workers were at the center on that day. Since the majority of the residents in the late

1980s and the 1990s were elderly and many had disabilities, staff members assisted the residents with their floats and costumes, and many of the workers participated and masked as well. Like the elderly men and women of the Aliyah Senior Citizens' Center in *Number Our Days* (Myerhoff 1979) who celebrated New Year's at noon on December 30 because midnight was too late for the elderly, and musicians can be hired at a lower rate the day before (1979: 10), the Carville residents adapted and improvised to meet the needs of their circumstances. For them, Mardi Gras on Friday was authentic and vital.

An important addition to the Carville Mardi Gras was the introduction of the Carville doubloons in the early 1980s.[4] Doubloons, metal coins imprinted with symbols of the Krewe or organization sponsoring the parade, were first minted and used as parade souvenirs or "throws" (that is, things for which spectators along the parade routes "beg" by yelling, "Throw me something, mister!") in the New Orleans Mardi Gras in 1960. In New Orleans and other urban Mardi Gras celebrations, the images on Mardi Gras doubloons are usually symbols of the "theme" for that year, often a topic of fantasy or mythology—Greek, Roman, and Egyptian are particularly popular. The Carville Krewe chose images that reflect both the place and the symbol of freedom from that place. According to Julia Elwood, as director of public

relations at Carville, the Patient-Staff Cultural Awareness Activities Committee at Carville decided on these
images for the doubloon. The committee first conducted
a survey at Carville and asked people to submit suggestions. The committee then chose the armadillo (with
Dasypus Novemcinctus, the scientific name for the
nine-banded armadillo, above the image and *Mardi Gras*
below) and the administration building. Elwood said
that these symbols "remind us of Carville, and they
are representative of Carville as we know it." She also
said that the administration building—the old Indian
Camp Plantation House—was there when the first leprosy patients arrived at Carville, via coal barge on the
Mississippi River, in 1894. Thus, it symbolizes the ori-
gins and continuity of Carville. The armadillo is a relatively new symbol. Elwood, who kept a figurine of an
armadillo on her desk, said that it symbolizes *hope* for
HD patients.

Only 2,500 Carville Mardi Gras doubloons were made
each year, and these were distributed to all the participants in the parade. Until 1998, the only date on the doubloons was 1921, the year the Carville hospital became
a Public Health Service hospital. The date was not
changed to indicate the year (an economic matter, since
a new die costs five hundred dollars), but the doubloons
were made in different colors each year—silver, gold,
green, and purple—repeating a color every four years.

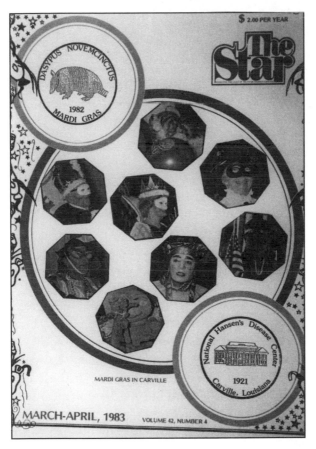

Cover of The Star, *Mardi Gras 1983, with images of the Carville doubloon. Courtesy of National Hansen's Disease Program.*

In 1998, the date on the doubloons (silver that year) was changed to 1894, the year the first seven patients arrived at Carville. As the doubloons were thrown out into the crowd, visitors and spectators engaged in friendly skirmishes trying to catch them in the air or to recover them from the ground. For older Carvillians, the doubloons encapsulate their lives. The armadillo symbolizes a fantasy or dream come true; it provided the means for discovery of a cure. With the Carville community, the images on the doubloons are examples of what Jack Santino calls "time-honored and meaning-drenched symbols," those cultural symbols that produce the most successful holiday creations (Santino 1995: 40). There is some irony, however, in their throwing these images out to spectators. The armadillo is believed by some in Louisiana to *cause* leprosy. There is also the unsubstantiated belief (or conjecture) that wild armadillos in Louisiana contracted leprosy because the leprosy-infected lab armadillos at the Gulf South Research Institute in New Iberia, Louisiana, escaped during a hurricane in the 1960s.[5] Because of these beliefs, outsiders sometimes attribute a different meaning and value to the armadillo as symbol. In this "meaning-drenched" inversion, the doubloon functions as another carnivalesque transgression.

Mardi Gras, wherever it is celebrated, is a kind of reversal, an opportunity to play with boundaries and experiment with identities, at least for the day. At Carville, it enabled the residents to be what they would like to envision themselves to be, and that included being able to celebrate as anyone else would. As Elwood said, "Mardi Gras is a very special time. People get into the spirit of things. There are some who actually go crazy." Most residents said they participated in the celebration because it was fun, something to look forward to, and this most certainly was an important reason for the continuation of the custom. But, more important, the Carville Mardi Gras, like other festivals ancient and modern, was a kind of "magical" ritual wherein participants were transformed, if only for a day. It is both a calendar festival with historical roots connected to the ecclesiastical calendar—a revelry before Lent—and a transformation of the people.

This element of transformation is basic to the performance of carnival. In the words of Victor Turner, "Truly carnival is the denizen of a place that is no place, and a time that is no time" (1987: 76). Louisiana writer Lyle Saxon gives his childhood memories of masquerading as devils for Mardi Gras in New Orleans: "I had the delightful feeling of being invisible—although the two devils were hailed from all sides—as though I had donned a magic cloak from some fairy tale, and were setting forth for strange adventures" (1988: 21). Samuel Kinser writes, "To enjoy the Carnival in New Orleans and Mobile demands suspension of disbelief. Tourist or native, one does best to enter with alacrity into a world of make-believe" (1990: 17).

Since the Carville Mardi Gras is based on the New Orleans celebration, New Orleans carnival fantasies and pretensions to king- and queenship roles have their counterparts in Carville. Role change and role reversal are important in many festivals. As de Caro and Ireland point out in regard to New Orleans Mardi Gras, "There is also the aspect of individual masking—that is, donning of costumes, though a mask or other method of face disguising is commonly a part of this—which allows people to act out private fantasies and to assume non-normal roles" (1988: 59). In Carville, however, the fantasies include not only royalty but the very state of being "normal." In Carville's Mardi Gras, the mask allows them to assume "normal" roles in the carnival; thus a masquerade becomes a means of achieving "normalcy" in a carnival context that is not possible for the physically deformed at any other times and that is often psychologically impossible for all HD patients. Julia Elwood came to Carville as a teenager, a former cheerleader at her high school in Texas. Her "Carville name" was Juliette Rivers, and she was Queen of the Mardi Gras in 1957. As a former patient whose appearance is completely unmarked by the disease, she said, "Even though you don't have the deformities, you still feel the stigma."

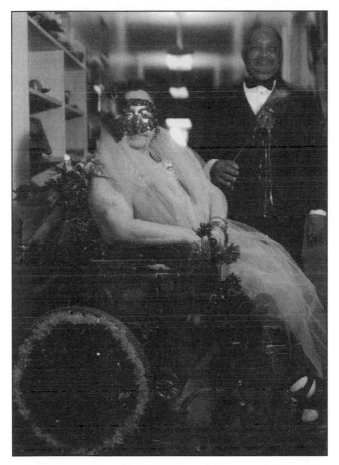

Queen and King, Mardi Gras at Carville, 1998. Photo by Jeffrey Braverman.

At Carville, the function of the mask was particularly important historically, for Mardi Gras was the one time when patients could hide their disfigurations in a socially sanctioned way—and when they, theoretically, could not be distinguished from "outsiders" or staff or "normal" people. On the occasion of the Mardi Gras in Carville in 1936, Sister Hilary Ross wrote in her journal, "With masks, when visitors came, they had nothing to fear. . . . We created our own happiness here." In the early Mardi Gras celebrations, the function of the masks to conceal the signs of leprosy on the face or simply to conceal one's identity from visitors or newspaper reporters and photographers was evident and clearly important. Visitors were not permitted to take photographs of residents on any other days. In the more recent Mardi Gras celebrations, concealing identity may still have been a function, but it was probably the least important. Very few residents at Carville in the last decades truly wanted or needed to conceal their identity. Much more important was the role of masks in transformation, a function that seemed to be intensified at Carville. Speaking in 1997 about her own experience of Mardi Gras at Carville, Julia Elwood said, "Wearing a mask does kind of free you from the everyday. . . . One year, I dressed as a clown, and I had the best time. No one knew who I was, so I did things I wouldn't have done otherwise. I danced, and I got the director to dance with me. It's a kind of freedom."

The mask can be a great equalizer. In medieval carnivals, masked peasants and noblemen mingled together. In Venice, Italy, it is said today that the mask allows one to "slip on a new skin." By hiding the face, masks negate the primary means of identification and recognition, but this negation also allows the possibility of something new—a transition, a transformation, however brief and temporary. Masks are almost invariably related to transition. David Napier suggests that "the mask is a means of transgressing boundaries because it provides an avenue of selective personification in manipulating certain recognized paradoxes" (1986: 17). Napier also points out that "all masks address some sort of transformation—some shift between planes of existence" (1987: 215). Richard Dorson contends, "Masks transform not only the physical appearance but also the psychic personality of the masquerader" (1982: 39).

Marianne Mesnil sees the mask as primarily an instrument of affirmation rather than disguise, and certainly this is true in most festivals. It functions, she says, to demarcate the break between "the order of being (the routine social order of a given society) and the order of seeming or representation" (1976: 12). Thus, the masked character indicates "the code by which his acts, expressions, and words must be interpreted. By simply wearing the mask, he indicates that he is representing something other than what he is as an individual, or even as a social being" (1976: 12).

J. C. Crocker suggests that "by donning masks—by hiding ourselves—we find our identity" (1982: 78). Although the process of transformation remains a mystery, masks are credited with magical powers, even in highly secularized maskings such as Mardi Gras. Victor Turner writes regarding carnival, ritual, and play in Rio de Janeiro, "One might even say that the masks, disguises, and other fictions of some kinds of play are devices to make visible what has been hidden, even unconscious" (1987: 77).[6]

At Carville, the function or role of masking seems to be greatly magnified. Transformation becomes heightened and intensified when "the place that is no place" and "the time that is no time" releases one from a very real place to which one was earlier confined by law solely on the basis of a stigmatizing disease. The mask disguises and conceals; more important, it also permits a powerful affirmation of the capacity for celebration with laughter and revelry. For those still haunted by popular delusions about leprosy and, indeed, allusions to "the living dead," the transformation from the carnival mask was a clear affirmation of life.

Carville was not a typical or autonomous folk community. Residents came from diverse backgrounds (ethnicity, religion, education, language, class, region). They all brought with them to Carville their memories of cultural

traditions, and they also adopted the local regional custom of carnival. For the majority of residents, Mardi
Gras was not a traditional celebration prior to their residence at Carville. But they shared certain beliefs, values, and survival strategies, particularly in dealing with
"one of the most meaning-laden of diseases" (Sontag
1989: 92) and with the resultant loss of control in their
lives. Most of all, they share the common experience of
dealing with what Erving Goffman calls "spoiled identity" (Goffman 1963). For many, whether they remained
at Carville or not, hiding aspects of their identity was
often felt to be imperative. Having to "masquerade" in
everyday life became a norm that was usually encouraged by physicians. Erving Goffman wrote in the early
1960s that the stigmatized individual "co-opts for his
masquerade" (that is, when he or she is hiding his or
her stigma) only those closest to him. Goffman says,
"Medical officials who discover a case of leprosy may
suggest that the new secret be kept among the doctors,
the patient, and his immediate family, perhaps offering
this discretion in order to ensure continued cooperation
from the patient" (1963: 95). In Mardi Gras at Carville,
the masquerade becomes an instrument of affirmation
for the patient residents. Instead of "hiding," they were
displayed—paraded for all to see, just like "normal"
people. As Roger Abrahams notes, "festivals provide
the occasion whereby a community may call attention

to itself and, perhaps more important in our time, its willingness to display itself openly" (Abrahams 1987: 181, emphasis in original).

Although Carville was admittedly a "culture of differentness," Carville's Mardi Gras seemed to fit Milton Singer's conception of cultural performance—those public events that encapsulate and display the values and symbols of a culture (Singer 1972: 70–75). In a celebratory manner, participants performed their group identity for themselves and for outsiders. As Stoeltje and Bauman point out, the messages embodied and enacted in cultural performances "give expression to the group's shared experience" (1988: 595). In this group, the central shared experience was difficult to display, celebrate, or even acknowledge in ordinary time. At the Carville Mardi Gras, they celebrated the triumph over their shared experience and literally threw out symbols of their shared identity in the form of the Carville doubloons. This open display of identity and cultural differentness was in itself an inversion of ordinary time for Carville residents, who typically had to masquerade their real identities and who traditionally did not call attention to themselves.

Does carnival serve the same function or does it have the same dynamics of role reversal, leveling, and so on, when the celebrators and participants are themselves (at least historically) the ultimate Others? Who or what was parodied in this masquerade? It was not a matter of class—since all classes were represented at Carville, as well as all races, genders, and educational levels. The Mardi Gras was also entirely within their own space. Although there were visitors and spectators, these were almost always people who had become, in a sense, "insiders" by the very fact of their being there. Other markers (race, gender, class, and religion) became largely irrelevant at Carville. The exclusionary force of the disease superseded any other dynamics. Perhaps it was really the *disease*, the stigma, that was turned on its ear, mocked, and inverted. But more important, it was the power of Mardi Gras to transform, to elevate, to overcome all other concerns, that worked its magic at Carville with a special intensity. In the context of Mardi Gras, the carnivalesque was doubly inverted, and the patients' humanity—normal, ludic, celebratory—was displayed. Their fear of the typical response of "outsiders" to the disease was dispelled. In the words of Mikhail Bakhtin, "Fear . . . is defeated by laughter" (1984: 47).

Carville's Mardi Gras was clearly not the Rabelaisian carnival described by Bakhtin, and indeed, many of Bakhtin's statements about carnivalesque grotesques seem particularly ironic if applied to Carville. However, some of Bakhtin's ideas about carnival do seem especially relevant to Carville. His following statement encapsulates the spirit and the effect of the Carville Mardi Gras: "Carnival with all its images, indecencies, and curses affirms the people's immortal, indestructible character. In the world of carnival the awareness of the people's immortality is combined with the realization that established authority and truth are relative" (Bakhtin 1984: 256).

{ 6 } "Under the Pecans"

HISTORY AND MEMORY IN THE GRAVEYARD AT CARVILLE

This is holy ground. I say that because there has been such suffering here.

—Sister Francis de Sales

The National Hansen's Disease Center at Carville had many of the marks and establishments of a typical community, and like other communities, it had a graveyard— a place to bury its deceased members. Unlike other communities, however, the shared identity of Carville residents was based on their shared medical diagnosis, Hansen's disease—or leprosy. For much of the twentieth century, patients diagnosed with leprosy were separated from society through legal quarantine and sent to live out their days at Carville, the National Leprosarium. Many stayed—even after death.

Memorials, markings, or gravestones serve a much more complex purpose than marking the location of a grave and identifying the individual buried there. They typically convey information about the person and his community of mourners. Often memorials comment on characteristics of the person and the mourners' relationships with that person. But they are also influenced by religion, ethnicity, regional geography, cultural identity, and the place of a person within the culture, for whatever reason. People express and communicate their relationship with the dead through material expressions—expressions literally carved in stone, concrete, and marble.

Cemeteries in general, and particularly in Louisiana, typically reflect cultural identities such as ethnicity, regionalism, and religious affiliation (Kniffen 1967, Nakagawa 1987). The early grave markers at Carville, with only initials, a first name, or a patient number, reflect the stigma of the disease that brought these people together and the need to keep their identities hidden, even in death. There was a cemetery at Carville almost from the beginning, when it was the "Louisiana Leper Home." Burial on hospital grounds began because patients in a leprosarium typically could not be buried in the church or public cemeteries in nearby towns or villages because of the objections of the public (see Enna and Byrd 1975). The bodies of deceased patients, however, could be returned for burial in their home-towns at the request and expense of their families. Residents of the Carville hospital were not buried in the nearby village of Carville. The original burial ground at the Carville hospital is now a courtyard in one of the quadrangles, surrounded by buildings, with a single marker, erected in 1921 and recording burials from 1895 to 1921. A stark reminder of Carville's past and the loss of identity of Carville's residents, it lists usually a first name, or the initials, or a patient number. (For details on the conflicting information on the grave markers and patient ledgers, see the appendix.)

When Carville became a U.S. government hospital in 1921, the government supplied standard national cemetery grave markers for the burial sites. Typically these were upright markers, forty-two inches long, thir-teen inches wide, and four inches thick. Each marker had a full name (first and last) engraved on it. However, it was almost never the real name of the person, since patients were encouraged to change their names when they entered Carville in order to protect their families. Each marker also had a patient number engraved below the name. Some families later added a more personal-ized marker to the grave. The new cemetery, opened in 1921 when the U.S. government took over, is located in a picturesque setting in a grove of pecan trees near Lake Johansen, in the back of the complex (the area farthest

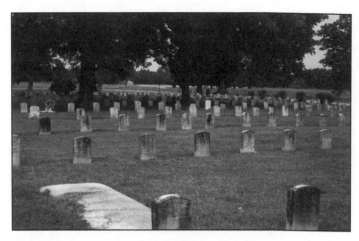

The "new" cemetery at Carville "under the pecans."

from the Mississippi River). Carville residents referred to the cemetery as "under the pecans," and they said "when I go under the pecans" to refer to their death.

The burial sites at Carville, one established in 1895 and the other in 1921, seem to be a reflection of the living history of Carville. Burial is typically in a place with meaningful ties to one's identity. For many, Carville seemed the most appropriate final resting place. For some, it is the place they came to against their wills and from which they never went "home" again. Those who never left were almost always buried there. Most who did leave and established a life elsewhere often chose to be buried elsewhere. For some, even some who had lives on the "outside" but kept their illness a secret, Carville is a place to come home to in death—the place where they did not have to masquerade, where they did not have to hide a significant part of their identity, where they did not have any secrets, except perhaps their real names. The graveyard at Carville and the tombstone monument in the quadrangle courtyard provide a reading of their trauma and loss of identity as well as the need for revisions of history and memory.

The symbolic resonance of a graveyard where "lepers" are buried is powerful, particularly given the history of society's treatment of leprosy patients. In the Middle Ages, leprosy patients were not only banned from living among the nonafflicted but could not even share a church or cemetery with them. In most parts of Europe, they were buried in separate cemeteries. In some parts of the Christian world, the Leper Mass was performed, with the living victim present, where priests filled an empty grave to symbolize their "death." They were then given a bell or clapper to warn others of their approach and their status as "the living dead." In thirteenth-century Europe, it was a civil crime for a leprosy patient to live among the healthy (Ell 302). Hawaiians refer to leprosy as "the separating sickness." W. S. Merwin's 1998 verse narrative of nineteenth-century Hawaii, *The Folding Cliffs*, describes leprosy as "the sickness that was a crime, and if somebody was accused of it that person would be taken away." Kalaupapa on Molokai is referred to as "the place they never came back from" (Merwin 120).

Even in the twentieth century in some parts of the world, customs for disposing of the corpses of victims of leprosy seem unbelievably inhumane. David Sapir discusses the practice of two customs of the Kujamaat Diola of southern Senegal: one the disposal of the corpse of a dead "leper," the other the disposal of the corpse of a hyena shot while hunting. He argues that "lepers" and hyenas are "natural symbols, that is, their interpretation or 'meaning' is transcultural and not specific to Kujamaat thought." (1981: 526–27). He gives a description of the two customs. A hyena shot in a hunt is given the ritual funeral and burial of an elder. He describes the "burying of a leper" as follows:

> When a leper with active leprosy dies, his corpse is attached by the hands and feet to a pole, as one would a pig or a large game animal. Then, covered with leaves, the body is rushed into the bush where it is dumped into a shallow grave that has been dug in advance. This is called *kabeten buying* (to throw away the corpse), in contrast to *etok buying* (to bury a corpse), as in a regular funeral (*nyikul*). For the ride out, a dog is tied to the leper's pole and corpse; it howls, yaps, and bites during the trip. At the grave, or just before it, the dog is dispatched by cutting its throat, and its body is

thrown into the bush. With the leper in his grave and
the dog in the bush, the carriers, along with the gravediggers, and still in a great hurry, fill the grave by kick-
ing at the dirt with their feet while facing away from
it. Such is their rush that they often fail to entirely
cover the body. On leaving the grave, the participants
run without looking back to wash themselves at a natural spring (as opposed to a man-made well). Throughout the entire proceeding the participants imitate the
noise of hyenas. The Kujamaat say, in effect, that the
carriers and gravediggers, until they are clean, and
the leper himself are like (and some would say are)
hyenas. (1981: 527)

Sapir goes on to say that "the care of lepers is the
responsibility of blacksmiths; the officiants at a leper's
funeral must all be blacksmiths, their agnates, or their
sisters' children" (1981: 527). Later, he says, "hyenas of
the area are of the spotted variety, which might recall
the sores and spots of a leper (though no informant volunteered this association)" (533). Both hyenas and
"lepers" arc thought to bc vchicles for witchcraft (535).

Eric Silla has described the death and burial of leprosy
patients among the Bobo and Dogon communities in late
twentieth-century Mali. Those with leprosy were buried
separately and often did not receive a proper burial.
He says:

Nothing emphasized the permanency of a leper's identity more than the practice among the Bobo and Dogon

communities of burying lepers in the bush away from "healthy" dead people. In such communities, leprous corpses often wound up inside cliffs, baobab trees, or termite mounds. For Sabari Sokoba, the prospect of such a burial caused him as much anguish and shame as the practices and belief which affected his more immediate day-to-day-life. . . . At most, communities would not wash the leper's body. (1998: 66–67)

Silla also says that often the bodies of leprosy patients were thrown into the bush, unprotected from wildlife, and that sometimes leprosy patients converted to Christianity because the White Sisters were kind and because they would then be buried in their cemetery (1998: 94).

While Carville's history is primarily a story in humanity and dignity in the treatment of Hansen's disease and its patients, the earliest patients experienced conditions not unlike those in Africa and medieval Europe. The earliest changes came with the arrival of the Daughters of Charity. Julia Elwood, in *With Love in Their Hearts*, the publication for the centennial anniversary of the Daughters of Charity at Carville, says of them:

They gave the patients at Carville hope that they would get a decent burial and that someone really cared. In a letter from Sister Beatrice [Sister Beatrice Hart, Sister Superior at Carville from 1896 to 1901] dated June 11, 1896, she writes: "Before we took charge of them they were thrown like dogs into the grave the same day they

died. I have insisted on a Christian burial as we understand it. Nothing short of a high Mass would satisfy
Father Colton. The Sisters sang. After Mass he made a
very feeling exhortation to those present, showing how
easy it is now for them to prepare for death, that in
Heaven there will be no deformity or disfigurement,
etc. The Libera was sung, the absolution was given and
the procession formed for the cemetery. Father Colton
leading. First came the men, next the women, last of
all the sisters. When we reached the grave, which Father
Colton helped the day before to open, he blessed it and
said the customary prayers. Then the body was low-
ered and we all came away, leaving the men (lepers) to
fill the grave. We felt we had buried the bodies of the
poor in the spirit of our Lord. Contrasting the reverent
care these bodies received with what was done to those
of their first associates who died here, has made a deep
impression upon the lepers and has, they say, taken
away all the sting of dying here." (Elwood 1996: 23–24)

In addition to patients and former patients, Daughters of
Charity who have served at Carville may also be buried
in the Carville cemetery. Grave markers for the Sisters
of Charity are in the shape of a cross. For example, the
graves of Sisters Zoe Schieswhol and Vincent Fleer are
side by side, each marked with a cement or concrete
cross. In an interview in 1998, Sister Francis de Sales
Provancher, eighty-one at the time and a Daughter of
Charity at Carville for over fifty years, said, "The only

thing I want is to be buried at Carville with my patients" (Roberts 1B).

In an article in *The Star* about the "bygone days" Ann Page talks about life at Carville before the U.S. government took over in 1921. Men and women were separated, by a fence or a wall, and even family members of the opposite sex could visit only once or twice a week in visiting booths along the dividing line. Funerals and burials (at that time in the cemetery in the present courtyard) were different. They were special "occasions." She says: "Funerals are usually synonymous with grief. With the exception of the immediate family, funerals here were occasions in those days. Sunday clothes were donned and the attendance was very large for the cemetery was the only place not separated by a fence or wall. At least you might steal a glance at some member of the opposite sex and that was something" (1944: 29). The dividing fences and walls that had separated the sexes for twenty-seven years were removed when Dr. Denney took charge for the U.S. Public Health Service.

Another change, of course, was the "new cemetery," located in a grove of pecan trees. Stanley Stein says in his 1963 memoir, *Alone No Longer*:

> The mossy oaks on the Carville reservation have always been symbols of the gayer moments of our existence. . . .
> The majestic pecan trees, on the other hand, have a somber connotation. Although they grow everywhere on

the old plantation, the tallest and the finest cast their
reverent shade on the little cemetery at the northerly
edge of Cottage Grove. And "under the pecans" has
become a Carville euphemism to describe the fate of a
patient who has gone the way of all flesh. (1963: 245)

According to a study on "Louisiana Necrogeography,"
trees are grown in 76 percent of Louisiana cemeteries. In
this study, however, pecan trees were not found to be a
typical tree grown in Louisiana cemeteries. According
to the study, the cedar (32 percent), live oak (14 percent),
pine (11 percent), crape myrtle (10 percent), and magno-
lia (7 percent) were the more popular trees in cemeteries
in south Louisiana (Nakagawa 117). Pecan trees are very
common in south Louisiana in general, and they are
found in some cemeteries. A classic Louisiana literary
example is beautifully depicted in Ernest J. Gaines's *A
Gathering of Old Men*. As the elderly black men wait in
the old graveyard where their people are buried, they
pick, crack, and eat pecans from the trees growing in the
graveyard. One of them says, "Graveyard pecan always
taste good" (1983: 47). This scene is based on the small
graveyard on River Lake Plantation (near New Roads)
where Gaines grew up, which does, indeed, have five
huge pecan trees. It is interesting to note in this context
a folk belief, at one time widely known in Louisiana,
that if a person plants a pecan tree, he or she will die the
first year the tree bears fruit.

"Under the pecans," in the "new" cemetery at Carville, every marker has two names—a first and last name. These names are usually their "Carville names," pseudonyms they took upon entering the hospital to protect their families. Some residents never changed their names and have their real names on the gravestones. Often these people had no contact with their home communities or families ever again after entering Carville. When the Louisiana Leper Home became the National Leprosarium in 1921, the system of numbering patients began anew with the number 1 for the first patient to enter Carville as a federal hospital. Thus the numbers in the new cemetery reflect this new numbering system, also starting over with Federal Register number 1.

The Carville cemetery is on the National Historic Register, part of Carville's historic district. People who have left Carville can request permission to be buried there, even if they no longer live there. Some of the people still living there said that if they left, they wanted to come back to be buried at Carville. Their families must pay for transportation of the body back to Carville.

There are about seven hundred graves and markers in the new cemetery. The U.S. government provides a National Cemetery type marker, but in some cases, the family provides a more personal marker. There are no special groupings of any kind in the cemetery. Although there was a time when black residents were

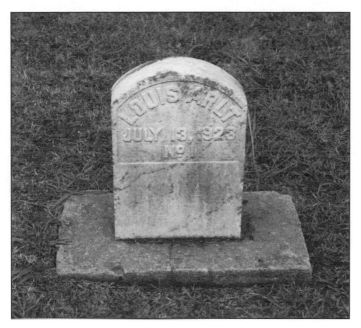

The grave marker of Louis Arlt, Patient #1, the first patient admitted to Carville after it became the National Leprosarium in 1921.

housed separately, the cemetery was completely integrated from the beginning. Pulitzer Prize-winning writer Rick Bragg, in a 1995 *New York Times* article on Carville, wrote: "Carville remains a place to hide and to be hidden. The headstones in the plain, military-like

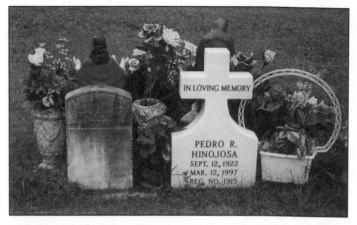

*The adjoining graves of Rafael Hinojosa (d. 1968) and Pedro
Hinojosa (d. 1997). Rafael's government marker gives only
the death date and registration number; Pedro's more recent
marker is personalized with "In Loving Memory" and
includes his date of birth.*

cemetery do not have much history on them. 'They
didn't want anyone to know, even in death,' Mrs.
Elwood said. 'Especially not in death.' Some have only
first names. Some have initials. Some are blank, except
for the patient's number. Some are lies written in
stone" (7A). Just as silence was a telling mode of nego-
tiation for the living, the metaphorical silence of the
early gravestones in Carville give us some indication of
what HD patients faced in their lives.

Each marker and gravesite in the "new" cemetery (under the pecans) has a story, often an untold story encrypted forever in stone. Whether the names on the stones are pseudonyms ("Carville names") or the real names of the deceased is often impossible to establish, since patients were not required to give their real names upon entering Carville.

The Carville cemetery sometimes reflects the complexity and irony of trying to both protect one's family and maintain one's sense of identity and dignity. Louis Boudreaux, former editor of *The Star*, his wife Kitty (Eloisa), and his brother (Emile, also a deceased patient) are all buried in the Carville cemetery in adjoining gravesites. All three changed their names upon entering Carville. As Louis Boudreaux said in a 1983 interview, patients were encouraged to change their names to protect their families. Though Louis and Kitty Boudreaux established identities at Carville and worldwide through *The Star* with those pseudonyms, their Carville names are not on their gravestones in the Carville cemetery. According to Kitty's sister Mary Ruth, Kitty's original gravestone did have her Carville name. Their mother, however, was upset upon seeing "Kitty Boudreaux" on her daughter's gravestone. Mary quoted their mother as saying, "My goodness—they had to change their names here, and now they have to go to the grave with those names" (Personal interview 2002). Louis Boudreaux

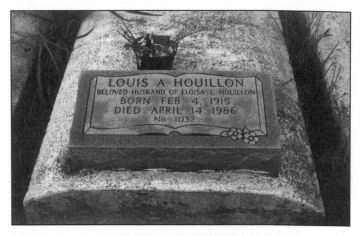

Grave of Louis A. Houillon (Louis Boudreaux).

decided then to replace the stone with her real name
(Eloisa Houillon), and his gravestone has his real name
as well (Louis Houillon).[1] Louis Boudreaux's in-ground
concrete vault has a personalized marble marker, but it
also has his patient number, "No. 1032."

The significance of the cemetery at Carville was evident when it was chosen as the site of a March 1999
protest by residents and others who wanted written
assurance that residents would not be forced to leave
Carville against their wills. About one hundred residents at the Hansen's Disease Center in Carville and
other supporters staged a demonstration to protest that

they may be once again forced to leave what had become home to them—with the closing of the center. In an event called "International Day of Dignity and Respect," a protest was held in the graveyard at Carville. It was organized by IDEA (Integration, Dignity, Economic Advancement), an international group that promotes understanding of Hansen's disease. Residents gathered, some in wheelchairs, some on bicycles and golf carts, at the front entrance and paraded to the graveyard where more than seven hundred Carville residents are buried. They carried hand-lettered signs of protest. A statement signed by residents read: "We were separated from our families and forced to create a new family. . . . Our husbands and wives and friends are buried in the cemetery here. If we are moved as planned, we will be uprooted and once again separated from our families. . . . To do this to us a second time is not only cruel, but unjust."

Though the U.S. Department of Health and Human Services had said residents would be allowed to remain, the protesters wanted something in writing. Anwei Skinsnes Law, who organized the event for IDEA, said, "We have a responsibility to people who live in these places not to uproot them for a second time." A small group of media and police were present. Though no written statement of assurance was forthcoming, the residents who chose to remain are being allowed to stay.

Several of them are helping with the National Hansen's Disease Museum, which officially opened on June 23, 2000.

It should be noted, however, that others who had remained at Carville until death even in the early twentieth century chose to be returned to their home communities for burial. This seems to have been more common when several family members had the disease and the fact of the illness was known among the patient's family and friends, though usually not by the entire community. For example, all five members of the New Iberia family who were patients at Carville were returned home for burial in the family tombs in Catholic cemeteries in Lafayette or in New Iberia. For the families, the death of someone with HD often brought to the forefront the continuing aspects of stigma associated with the disease. Johnny P. Harmon writes in his memoir, *King of the Microbes*, "On November 4, 1941, my dearly beloved brother lost his final battle with Hansens" (1996: 63). He goes on to say:

> I was at work when my father called and gave me the news of Elmo's death. . . . My father made the necessary arrangements to bring Elmo's body home for burial. The Government would have buried him in the hospital cemetery but we wanted to bring him home. In those days, if a casket was removed from the hospital, it had to be sealed. That rule is no longer in effect. So, we brought home a sealed casket. There was a large

crowd at Elmo's funeral but no one got to see him. I did
not see them put my brother in that sealed box but I
feel sure they did. Of course, it is possible that we
brought home an empty box. (64)

The sanitary codes of 1911, specifying the rules for
burial and removing bodies, are mentioned in the journals of the Daughters of Charity and cited by Enna and
Byrd (1975): The bodies of patients with a number of
diseases including leprosy had to be thoroughly disin-
fected before being accepted for transfer.

Though modern medicine has provided a cure for the
disease and Carville is no longer open as a treatment center, the effects of the stigma are not totally gone. Leprosy
patients today are still forced to protect their personal
identities. Said a contemporary leprosy sufferer in
Athens, Greece, "The story of leprosy sufferers as living
dead must finally come to an end" (Drakos 1997). The
graveyard and grave markers at Carville have important
meanings. They implicitly provide signs through which
the trauma and endurance of the last group of people
banished from society because of an illness can be interpreted and understood.

David Sloane, in a study of American cemeteries, said:
"The American cemetery is a window through which we
can view the hopes, fears, and designs of the generation
that created it and is buried within it" (1991: 6). This
assumes that the agency and decision-making power to

create the cemetery were possessed by members of the group who would be buried there. That was not the case with the Carville cemetery, or in general, with any national cemetery. The Carville cemetery, however, in many ways reflects the role and status of those buried there—both patients in a "leprosarium" and human beings with a sense of their own dignity and need for identity.

Richard Meyers in *Ethnicity and the American Cemetery* said, "cemeteries are far more than merely elements of space sectioned off and set aside for the burial of the dead: they are, in effect, open cultural texts, there to be read and appreciated by anyone who takes the time to learn a bit of their special language" (1993: 3). This "special language" of the Carville gravestones is often the absence of language. The silence that Carville patients felt they had to observe in life outside of Carville is reflected in the silence of their gravestones.

Many HD patients and former patients now do speak out through their personal narratives. For most of those buried in the Carville graveyard, their gravestones tell their stories. The Carville graveyard also tells us about the effects of ignorance and fears of the larger society that set up such an institution—and condemned its citizens to a life of exile within their own country solely on the basis of a medical diagnosis.

{ 7 } Remembering Leprosy

POSTMEMORY AND THE CARVILLE LEGACY

It is not what we have lost that matters most, but what we choose to do with what we have left.

—STANLEY STEIN

G. W. Long Hansen's Disease Center at Carville officially closed in 1999. At the same time, the National Hansen's Disease Program was relocated to Summit Hospital Complex in Baton Rouge, Louisiana. The closing of the center at Carville was followed a year later by the opening of the National Hansen's Disease Museum on the same site on June 23, 2000. The founders established the museum with the wish "to assure that the 104 years of mankind's history that took place here is not lost."[1]

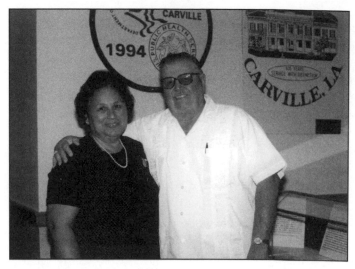

Julia and Ray Elwood, at the official opening of the National Hansen's Disease Museum at Carville, June 23, 2000.

While Carville is no longer the site of the National Hansen's Disease Program, the effects of diagnosis and compulsory isolation at Carville are far from over. Many of the people who were confined to Carville by quarantine laws have passed away. Others are now elderly patients being treated in the center in Baton Rouge for age-related illnesses. Some who entered voluntarily after quarantine laws ended, such as the Elwoods and José Ramirez, are now spokespersons for Hansen's disease education.

An even larger group of people are still being affected by the trauma of Carville. These are the children, grand-children, and even great-grandchildren of people who lived through the stigma of being diagnosed with lep-rosy. A diagnosis of leprosy affected the entire family. The patient was taken to Carville, but the family was left to mourn the loss, almost always in silence—public silence, if not private silence.[2] The second-generation memories, once silenced, are now being voiced by the children, grandchildren, great-grandchildren, and other relatives of former Carville residents.

In a study of second-generation memory of the Holocaust, "Projected Memory," Marianne Hirsch fur-ther develops her concept of *postmemory*. She uses the term *postmemory* "to describe the relationship of chil-dren of cultural or collective trauma to the experiences of their parents, experiences that they 'remember' only as the stories and images with which they grew up, but that are so powerful, so monumental, as to constitute memories in their own right" (1999: 8). In *Family Frames*, Hirsch says that "postmemory is distinguished from memory by generational distance and from history by deep personal connection" (1997: 22). She goes on to say: "Postmemory characterizes the experience of those who grow up dominated by narratives that preceded their birth" (1997: 22). While Hirsch developed this con-cept based on the children of Holocaust survivors, focusing on the function of family photographs, she believes it can apply to other second-generation memories of trauma. The concept of postmemory can be used as a frame to understand and appreciate the second-generation memories of trauma for family members of patients diagnosed with leprosy and forced by law to leave their homes for Carville.

For second-generation Holocaust survivors, Hirsch points out that photographs serve as a form of evidence to "affirm the past's existence" (1997: 22–23). While Hirsch uses photographs as catalysts or sites of postmemory, letters from patients at Carville can function in the same way as a form of evidence of the past's existence. Along with personal narratives, letters from patients at Carville give tangible evidence to their descendants of the traumatic family experiences that inevitably affected their lives.

Possibly the most extensive collection of letters from Carville is in the possession of the Landry and Manes families of New Iberia, Louisiana. The letters were written by two brothers, Norbert and Edmond Landry, to members of their family, mainly their parents, Lucy and Terville Landry. The letters of Edmond Landry to his wife, Claire Landry, are not in the collection and are thought by their daughter to have been burned or otherwise destroyed. Norbert Landry was a patient from 1919 to 1924, and Edmond Landry was a patient from 1924 to 1932. Both died at Carville. Their three younger siblings were all later patients at Carville, until the last one died in 1977. The collection of letters is now in the possession of Leonide Landry Manes, daughter of Edmond Landry. At present, two family members in Louisiana are working on academic projects involving the letters. Claire Manes, daughter of Leonide Manes and granddaughter of Edmond Landry, is a Ph.D. student in English and folklore at University of Louisiana at Lafayette. Christopher Manes, grandson of Leonide Manes (son of John Manes and nephew of Claire Manes) and great-grandson of Edmond Landry, completed his M.A. in English and creative writing at the University of Louisiana at Lafayette and is now a doctoral student at University of Texas at Dallas. Another family member, living in Georgia, is working on a play based on the letters. Members of the Landry and Manes families have shared some of their responses to their own postmemory of Carville and the letters written and sent from Carville.

In *Alone No Longer*, Stanley Stein says the turning point for him following his admittance to Carville "was probably Gabe Michael's misfortune. Gabe was the only altruistic character I had so far met at Carville. . . . He was the man who had founded the patients' canteen and was managing it without salary" (1963: 53). Stein says that the political heart of Carville was the patients' canteen (61). Though Gabe Michael died the year after

Stanley Stein came to Carville, he had inspired Stein to become an activist.

Leonide Landry Manes, daughter of Edmond G. Landry (alias Gabe Michael), talked about her father in an August 2000 interview with me (along with her daughter and grandson). Mrs. Manes says that her mother never talked about her father's illness. She said, "And I've told them all—it wasn't that she was ashamed of where he was, but—because she never would use the fictitious name. She addressed him as Edmond. She never used Gabe Michael. It wasn't that. It was to protect us." She says that her mother's response of silence, she thinks, was an attempt to keep the children from being hurt. Mrs. Manes said also that her mother didn't explain what the disease was until she was older. She said:

> When we were older—but she didn't talk much, but she then told us what it was. But, she didn't—as I tried to explain to Paul—I think she was trying to keep us from being hurt. Because you see, people in New Iberia didn't understand what it was either. There weren't a lot of people from here who had it.
>
> And I told you this [to Claire]—I was going to the post office one morning ('cause even at six years old you could walk from my house to Main Street safely). And I went in front of a place we used to call the "yellow quarters." They were yellow houses, rent

houses, and the people sat on their porches from morning till night. And I remember I went past and they didn't realize that I would understand a little French, and they said in French that I was the girl whose Daddy had that bad disease. Now, I'm sure if you had asked them what the bad disease was they wouldn't have known—but that's how things went. I can remember one incidence that happened to me—I was in the fifth grade at school, and a girl—I still see that girl today, and she's very nice to me [Claire: "She'd better be"]—Well, she caught a good spanking. But, she, it was at lunch recess, and she said—we were all in a group—and she said, "Your daddy's at the crazy house." She could have said, "the insane asylum" and I believe I would have accepted it. But she said, "Your daddy's at the crazy house." Kids can be cruel. And I walked away, and I was crying. And somebody went and told the principal what she did. (Personal interview 2000)

Mrs. Manes also said that she learned about leprosy primarily through reading. When she brought letters to the post office, she saw the address "Carville, Louisiana." She said, "And then one day, I saw an article in the paper. I saw an article about Carville, and they named the illness—leprosy. And because my mother was reticent, I guess we were reticent with her, too. . . . And ah, so I looked up the word, and I learned what it was" (Personal interview 2000).

Mrs. Manes talked about a later incident in her life as well, which she remembers in detail:

> I remember one incident in my life that did affect me. But, like everything else, you just didn't say it at the time. I tell my children, I have a tendency to be a little stand-offish with people. And I'm sure it's the things I held back. You know, if you—still, I don't know if I would have given this interview if MaMa was still living.
>
> But, I had a friend—when in college she was tutoring a boy, and his mother told her one day that she didn't like the idea of her associating with me. (Of course, she never let her go either. I mean, she could have—) And, ah, she said because her father is sick, and he has a disease that's very contagious." Of course, she didn't know. She asked me, she said, "Is that true?" I said, "Yea, it's true." And he died shortly after that. And I said, "But, it's not really that contagious." She believed me, and she was all right with it. But I said, "It's not as contagious as that lady thinks." I said, "They don't know what causes it." Well, they did know it was a bacillus, but they didn't know how it was passed on. (Personal interview 2000)

Perhaps the most traumatic memories for Mrs. Manes are her recollections of the day her father left for Carville and the circumstances of his brief returns for visits to family in New Iberia:

> I remember the day he left. My grandmother always lived with us. She had been there when Daddy and my uncle

went off to war—and she moved in with us. My mother's
mother. My father's mother lived out [in the country]. I
stayed with my grandmother, and they drove off. Kissed
us all and went off. And, ah, you see, he volunteered.
Well, he volunteered because Dr. Sabatier told him if he
did, they didn't have to take him off in shackles. I think
Dr. Sabatier must have explained that to him at some
point—that if he didn't go willingly—since he had been a
diagnosed case and it had gone through the Iberia Parish
Board of Health, yes, he would have to leave anyway. Or
it would be a matter of going "on the run" somewhere
else, and he did go—with my grandfather and one of my
grandfather's brothers. One thing I remember—they had
his luggage (it wasn't a great deal because they didn't
need a great deal) on the side of the car, and I don't know
what happened to it, but they lost it. So they had to trace
their way back—almost all the way and then go back.
And in those days—it's not a bad trip today—but in
those days you had to go all the way to Opelousas, across
the old bridge and back. It was a hard trip.

And Daddy was gone. He was there for eight years,
and in those eight years, he came home twice. But
only—his mother was sick both times. One time she
had an appendectomy operation. Not the first time—
but the second time. And he came under armed
guard—and that's something I've never forgiven them
for, and I never will. (Personal interview 2000)

At that time, patients did not yet get regular leave
time from Carville. They were allowed short leave

because of illness or death in the family, but they were escorted by armed guards, just as prisoners are escorted under armed guard to attend the funeral of a close relative. Mrs. Manes explained:

> But they came with their leggings and their khaki pants and their stiff military round brim caps and the gun on the side. And you know—I was across the street—we didn't know he was coming—and when the car drove up, it scared me to death. But, the lady knew what it was, and she told me, she said, "That's your daddy." And she said, "You can go home to your mama." So, I crossed over—but, ah—they didn't stay at the house. He went to his mother's house. You see, there was something about children. . . . But, ah, he stayed, I think, overnight, and went back after his mother was okay. He went back the next day. But both times, it was under guard. And he was not one—I don't think—who would have run away. I know he wasn't the happiest person in the world while he was there, and I think it was being separated from his family. There were a lot of reasons, I know. You give up your life, really. And in those days—you see now, and even when Albert and Marie were there—not when they went but after they were there a year or two—there was—sulfone drugs were found, and then it was all right. But, at that time, there was no hope. (Personal interview 2000)

While these memories are being expressed in personal narratives by Mrs. Manes, the letters from Edmond

Landry and his brother Norbert Landry along with her narratives are tangible sources of postmemory for her children and grandchildren. They have used these as the basis for scholarly research, narratives, and poetic expressions of their own.

Both Claire Manes and Christopher Manes are in the process of writing about their family members, based in particular on the letters and their own postmemory. The encrypted narratives and the silences shaped their understanding of Carville and of their family. While both Claire Manes and Christopher Manes were students at the University of Louisiana at Lafayette, the Landry family gave me access to the letters. Since they will be using these letters as the basis for their own ongoing scholarship, I will refer only to parts of the letters that they have already cited in their presentations or publications. The letters show the thoughts and the anguish of leprosy patients, before the term *Hansen's disease* was in use. I am struck with the force of some of the letters—they have none of the amelioration or the hindsight perspective of the memories of survivors of HD in the late twentieth century. The writers of the letters, at least at times, knew there was little hope that they could ever be cured or would ever leave Carville alive. Yet they were able to find some meaningful, though certainly compromised, way to live their lives.

Claire Manes, as a third-generation survivor, has personal memories of family members who were patients at Carville during her lifetime and whom she visited at Carville, though of course she has only second-generation postmemory of her grandfather. She presented her own perspective along with quotes from the family letters and letters from government officials in her presentation, "In His Own Hand—The Correspondence of Edmond G. Landry from Carville, Louisiana," at the Louisiana Folklore Society Meeting, Lafayette, April 5, 2003:

> On October 3, 1924, Dr. Oscar Dowling, president and executive officer of the Louisiana State Board of Health wrote to Dr. W. F. Carstens, the chief health officer for Iberia parish (quote): "Dr. O. E. Denney Medical Officer in Charge of the United States Marine Hospital #66 . . . authorizes me to have Mr. E. G. Landry, leper, 33, male, married, sent forward." Thus began a week of official correspondence leading ultimately to Edmond G. Landry's voluntary incarceration in the national leprosarium in Carville, Louisiana. . . .
>
> Edmond Landry was my grandfather. He entered Carville in October of 1924 and died there in December 1932, thirteen years before I was born. I grew up with silence surrounding him. I knew that he had "died in a hospital" and that he had had leprosy, a truth I learned painfully when I was nine or ten. However, the truth that I absorbed most keenly was that we did not talk about him. On the few occasions when I ventured to ask about him I would experience a silence filling the

room and I would hear the same mantra repeated,
"He died of kidney disease in a hospital." (Claire
Manes 2003)

Silence seems to be an important formative influence
on her postmemory of the family narrative. What
marked the family narratives for her was the absence
of story. She uses the collection of letters as a source
for reconstructing a family narrative.

In his essay "Regarding Carville: The Letters of
Norbert and Edmond Landry," Christopher Manes also
looks at the letters written by the two brothers to their
families from 1919 to 1924 (Norbert) and 1924 to 1932
(Edmond). Manes says that the letters "transform historical facts and politics concerning leprosy, now better
known as Hansen's disease, into human experience"
(2003: 325). He says that the letters show that the
brothers turned to strategies for coping—religious faith
and prayer for Norbert and activism and altruism for
Edmond. Edmond refers to himself as "just a leper," and
he deplores the lack of any real progress in the treatment
of the disease. In an interview with Sarah Spell Johnson,
Chris Manes said, "I don't think my family was ashamed
of them or ashamed of the disease. But to have had the
lives of an entire generation just stripped away from
them was too painful to discuss" (Johnson 2001: 1B).

Christopher Manes's chapbook, *Regardez*, is a
collection of poetic responses to the letters of his

great-grandfather and great-great-uncle from Carville, as well as responses to the memories of his grandmother. His M.A. thesis expands on these responses. In the poems, Manes uses lines from the letters as inspirations for his poetic responses, written in Edmond Landry's voice as he addresses his wife, Claire Landry, in his letters:

> *Claire, I don't expect you to understand.*
> *Here I am human again,*
> *less a leper today than I've been.*

In another poem, Manes reflects poetically on the writings of Edmond Landry to his wife in 1927, at the time of the impending flood of the Mississippi River in Louisiana (the "great flood of '27"). Using information in the family letters as a basis, he imagines how Edmond may have written to his wife:

> *Claire, the river situation is worse.*
> *The levee has become indifferent*
> *And I am afraid the rest of the world with it.*
> . . .
> *The sisters tell me to keep my faith . . . Trust*
> *But I don't know, Claire,*
> *The authorities have a boat in front the*
> *big house for their use.*
> . . .

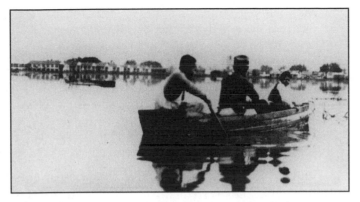

High water at Carville, Mississippi River flood of 1927.
Courtesy of National Hansen's Disease Program.

This poem is especially forceful in light of an interview I conducted with Sister Laura Stricker in January 1984. Sister Laura came to Carville in 1925. She worked at Carville as a medical records librarian and pharmacist until 1971, and then she stayed there as a retired sister until 1984. She said:

> In 1927, we had the high water, and we had to use
> sandbags to hold the water. They had a barge out there,
> and they had men on the barge all night long. And
> if the levee would break, they were supposed to bring
> the patients out of the hospital and on to the barge.
> There were handicapped people who couldn't walk

> and some were blind, and if they would have had to get
> them out there—I don't think they would have made
> it. . . . We had about 350 patients, I think. (Personal
> interview 1984)

This interview was done with Sister Laura long before I
knew of the existence of the Landry family letters, so
clearly Sister Laura's response was an objective evalua-
tion of the situation that undoubtedly corroborates
Mr. Landry's concerns and validates that the patients,
in spite of what they were being told by the authorities,
had serious cause for alarm about their situation during
the flood.

Christopher Manes also was inspired poetically by
his grandmother's memory of the funeral of her uncle
(Chris's great-great-uncle) Norbert Landry in 1924.
Mrs. Manes was five years old at the time. Her own
father, Edmond Landry, would enter Carville later that
year. In an interview with Chris, when he asked her,
"What is your first memory?" she said: "At Norbert's
funeral, the coffin was opened. Aunt Adrienne picked
me up off the ground. I was only five then. She lifted me
on her shoulder and made me look at his remains. She
shouted, 'Regardez' " (Christopher Manes 2003: 29). This
is Chris Manes's beautifully moving and poetic response,
giving voice and interpretation to an event in his

family's history that occurred almost six decades before his birth, but whose force continues to resound:

Regardez

Aunt Adrienne lifted her forward
and shouted Regardez
She wanted her niece to remember that
no matter what was to come,
no matter what anyone
would ever tell her
He was human in the coffin.

What Leonide remembered
was that the sound of Regardez
echoed out the casket
as if the dead had spoken it.
(Christopher Manes 2003. Used with permission)

Here in Chris Manes's words, we have a summary of what must be remembered about HD patients or anyone else affected by illness: they are people. They are part of about 5 percent of the world's population who lack a genetically determined natural immunity from the HD bacillus. They are human beings, like everyone else, who happen to have a bacterial disease.

Appendix A

CARVILLE DEATH RECORDS ON CEMETERY MARKER

The numbers and dates given on the memorial grave marker and information recorded in a Carville patient ledger dated August 31, 1897, are in disagreement. According to information on the bronze grave marker memorial, the original seven patients who came to Carville in December 1894 were:

> J. A. Greaud (No. 1, died 1906) [Carville ledger records death of patient No. 1 as 1896*]
> H. Collins (No. 2, died 1896)
> J. Mocklin (No. 3, died 1904)
> R. L. Fish (No. 4, died 1901)
> J. Eickinger (No. 5, died 1902)
> Mrs. Schultz (No. 6, died 1895)
> ? (No. 7)
> C. Mertz (No. 8, died 1902)

In the "List of Patients in Leper Home of La. to date Aug. 31, 1897," reprinted in Elwood's 1994 centennial publication, no names are given; patients are listed only by number. A girl patient, Clara Mertz, is listed in a December 2, 1894, *New Orleans Daily Picayune* article as one of the seven original patients transported to Carville in

December 1894, but the bronze grave marker lists a C. Mertz as patient "No. 8." However, patient No. 8 is listed in the 1897 ledger as a twenty-nine-year-old male, and patient No. 7 is a twenty-four-year-old female (presumably Clara Mertz). It is clear that the numbers on the grave memorial plaque do not identify the same patients as corresponding numbers on the 1897 ledger. The complete information that appears on the bronze marker erected in the courtyard, site of the original graveyard, in 1922 is as follows:

Erected by
The United States of America
In Memory of Deceased Patients of
This Hospital June 1922

1895

NO. 10   J. D.

NO. 12   C. COLLET

NO. 6   MRS. SCHULTZ

1896

NO. 2   H. COLLINS

NO. 11   J. BROWN

NO. 29   T. VOLMER

1897

NO. 30   H. SHERMAHOUR

NO. 24   TINA

NO. 16   E. RUSSEL

NO. 32   H. BERGER

[**1898**–None listed]

1899

NO. 38   MRS. A. CARTER

NO. 40   C. NEWMAN

1900

NO. 36   J. LANG

NO. 48   G. HUNTZINGER

NO. 18   F. GREAUD

NO. 20   E. JOSEPH

1901

NO. 4   R. L. FISH

NO. 25   MRS. K. LEE

NO. 9   W. BREEN

1902

NO. 13   FRANK GEX

NO. 49   H. GIBBONS

NO. 8   C. MERTZ

NO. 58   A. MILLER

NO. 5   J. EICKINGER

NO. 23   NINA

NO. 17   C. JACKO

1903

NO. 35	R. OLLIE
NO. 59	M. KING
NO. 52	JULIE
NO. 75	J. FORESTAL
NO. 39	J. BOTHMAN
NO. 37	ROSINA
NO. 21	M. JOSEPH
NO. 56	B. JONES

1904

| NO. 72 | MRS. KROMER |
| NO. 3 | J. MOCKLIN |

1905

| NO. 31 | J. WILLIAMS |
| NO. 96 | MRS. RAYMOND |

1906

NO. 98	H. O.
NO. 1	J. A. GREAUD
NO. 34	H. R. HAUG

1907

| NO. 111 | W. B. |

1908

| NO. 66 | PAT |

1909

NO. 105	J. L.
NO. 77	EUGENE
NO. 109	MRS. JONES

NO. 74	A. GREY
NO. 114	ODETTE
NO. 33	MAY

1910

NO. 116	A. SIMEON
NO. 143	T. D.
NO. 140	A. ROUEL
NO. 67	M. KEHOE
NO. 136	D. M.
NO. 86	J. WATSON
NO. 142	SOPHY
NO. 68	GASTON
NO. 85	MRS. KLIBERT
NO. 113	EMMA
NO. 152	J. Z.

1911

| NO. 176 | A. CONGO |

1912

NO. 157	M. BROWN
NO. 178	F. B.
NO. 88	DAVE KERN
NO. 27	FERDINAND
NO. 183	JOHN SEABOLD

1913

NO. 55	MARIE ROSS
NO. 71	ADOLPH
NO. 76	A. BRYANT
NO. 87	MARIE
NO. 93	MRS. OLIKE

NO. 100 J. PFEIFFER
NO. 135 OLIVER

1914
NO. 104 TEDDY
NO. 126 MARY JOSEPH
NO. 137 LEON

1915
NO. 117 J. MARTINA
NO. 42 A. BORNE
NO. 210 M. BRYANT
NO. 156 EVA
NO. 41 EDWARD
NO. 60 WALTER
NO. 188 D. F.
NO. 193 ISABEL
NO. 217 BULLINGER
NO. 112 A. BROWN

1916
NO. 226 JERRY
NO. 147 GEO. WASHINGTON
NO. 127 FRANK WEITZEL
NO. 207 J. S.
NO. 110 PETER CARROLL
NO. 102 HANK
NO. 83 D. BONVILLIAN
NO. 134 MRS. MILLER
NO. 235 OLIVE TOUCHET
NO. 78 W. F.
NO. 118 PETER BUCK

NO. 141 WAUKEE
NO. 174 MRS. CLEMM
NO. 108 MRS. ELIZA RUTH

1917
NO. 198 JACOB JONES
NO. 187 ADAM WARREN
NO. 162 WILLIE
NO. 145 MRS. TRAHAN
NO. 15 ROSIE

1918
NO. 286 P. KLING
NO. 269 VIOLA CAULEY
NO. 247 H. PARKER
NO. 253 MAY
NO. 73 JOE ALBRIER
NO. 255 MR. EMILE
NO. 259 MRS. J. KLIBERT
NO. 61 ARTHUR

1919
NO. 209 JOE ROCHESTER
NO. 146 J. M.
NO. 262 JOE PERRY
NO. 154 M. H.
NO. 107 ALMA

1920
NO. 47 JOHN CALLAHAN
NO. 63 MARTINE
NO. 311 MRS. A. F.
NO. 144 GERTRUDE

NO. 335	MRS. M. F.	NO. 64	E. OLSEN
NO. 192	LILLY	NO. 77	LUCIEN
NO. 175	PAUL	NO. 91	EMILE
NO. 305	JULES	NO. 20	EPHRAIM
		NO. 23	J. FRANK
1921		NO. 27	J. GRAY
NO. 69	OWENS	NO. 29	J. MARTIN
NO. 30	W. H.		
NO. 114	THOMAS	**1922**	
NO. 28	H. R. H.	NO. 158	A. GROVEN

Appendix B

Welcome to a community unlike any other in the world, many of whose residents experienced two opposite emotional extremes—one is extraordinary physical suffering, separation of families, endless psychological stress, emotional breakdown, and another is security, healing and comfort—a haven—a place to hide.

Leprosy, or Hansen's disease, has traditionally and historically carried an emotionally damaging stigma. Through the ages there has been widespread misconception about what has been called history's most dreaded disease. The ancient scourge can cause disfigurement, paralysis, disability, loss of sensation, and mental anguish. Persons affected by leprosy have experienced ostracism, imprisonment, and rejection for no other reason than because they were diagnosed with this most misunderstood of diseases.

Numerous physicians, therapists, nurses, scientists and support staff have collaborated in the training, rehabilitation, education, research, and treatment at the Center through the years. This is the place where several medical breakthroughs were discovered beginning with the sulfones in 1941, the first effective treatment of leprosy.

Stories of tragedy, breakups, joy, sadness, loneliness, self-sacrifice, love, hate, misery, isolation, companionship, hope, injury, faith, outrage, despair, success, doubt, hopelessness, anger, and imprisonment make this place a unique American true story about individuals caught in a microbes versus medicine battle unmatched anywhere.

Notes

Chapter 1. Carville, Leprosy, and Real People

1. See also Brody 1974 and Richards 1977 for more on medieval leprosy. For more on the early history of hospitals for the isolation of leprosy patients, see chapter 4, "Hospitals as Segregation and Confinement Tools: Leprosy and Plague," in Risse 1999 (167–229).

2. Over the next century, 112 Daughters of Charity were assigned to Carville. Among them were Sister Hilary Ross, who came to Carville in 1922 and served for thirty-seven years, first as a pharmacist and then as a biochemist. Sister Hilary's unpublished journal is the source of much information about Carville. Sister Laura Stricker came to Carville in 1925 and served for forty-seven years as a medical records librarian and pharmacist. Sister Laura also directed theatrical productions and music at Carville. Many, like Sister Francis de Sales Provancher, Sister Rose D'Alfonso, Sister Margaret Brou, and Sister Francis Louviere, stayed at Carville as volunteers after their retirement. For more on the Daughters of Charity at Carville, see *With Love in Their Hearts: The Daughters of Charity of St. Vincent de Paul, 1896–1996*, a Carville Centennial Publication edited by Julia Elwood.

3. See Kalisch 1972 for more on "The Strange Case of John Early."

4. For more information, see February 2001 issue of the science journal *Nature*.

5. For more on Carville's history, see Gussow 1989 and Calandro 1983. For more on the history of leprosy, see Trautman 1985.

6. Julia Rivera Elwood addresses the issue of Louisiana's role in the care and treatment of leprosy patients in the 1996 publication

honoring the Centennial of Daughters of Charity at Carville. In a section entitled "Kudos to Louisiana," she says:

> It may be odd that Louisiana harbored the only leprosarium on the American Continent. The reason was that, historically, Louisiana, beyond all other states combined, pioneered in the study, treatment, and suppression of the malign disease. To the Pelican State in a large part belongs the credit for the relative rarity of leprosy in our country at the present time. On Louisiana soil the major battles against the disease have been fought ever since the days of the Spanish occupation when Governor Ulloa, in 1766, established the first lazaretto, or quarantine leper colony, at Balize, about 80 miles below New Orleans. [1996: 51]

7. Since quarantine laws were established by individual states, it is difficult to establish an exact date when leprosy was no longer subject to quarantine in the United States. Patients from other states on official leave had to get permission to travel through any state en route. Most states prohibited leprosy patients from traveling on public transportation. By 1960, most patients were admitted to Carville on a voluntary basis.

8. Though I have heard that there was a "Colored House" at one time, it does not seem that races were segregated in any other way. According to Tanya Thomassie, a longtime staff member and current director of public relations, the assignment to a specific house was based on "similarities in culture, education, and nationality, rather than racial divisions" (Thomassie 2004). She also said that languages, food, and music preference were often deciding factors, as well as simply the requests of the patients themselves. It should be noted that a very small percentage of patients at Carville were African American. In her 1994 publication on the Carville centennial, Julia Elwood quotes an unidentified source on statistics at Carville in the 1950s, when there were about four hundred patients:

> About 40% of the patients are foreign born, with Mexicans predominating. Next to the Mexicans come Chinese, and then Greeks. Of the

Notes { 193 }

American born patients, few are negroes. Leprosy is not prevalent
among the negroes in the United States, but when they do contract
it they become very bad cases. All in all, there are representatives of
26 states and 20 nationalities. (Elwood 1994: 46)

Chapter 2. "An Exile in My Own Country"

1 Culbertson deals with acute trauma and survivors of physical
violence, and her theories are not wholly applicable to the kind of
trauma suffered by HD patients. For example, recovered memory is
not a part of HD patients' experience. The memory of leprosy may
be silenced, but it is never totally repressed. But Culbertson's ideas
about bodily memory do have some relevance for those who lived in
what may be called a chronically traumatized state.

2. Even before Carville became the National Leprosarium, it was
not truly a secret place. When John Early entered Carville in 1918, it
received national attention. Early was a vocal and controversial leprosy patient as well as a notorious absconder, who testified before the
U.S. Congress and greatly influenced legislation establishing Carville
as a federal facility. While Carville may not have been widely known
nationally, it was clearly not a secret in Louisiana. Daily tours were
given, and by 1968, over 13,000 people toured Carville. When I was a
student at Louisiana State University in the early 1960s, sororities,
fraternities, and other student organizations visited Carville at
Christmas and other times during the year, as student groups would
visit hospitals, "old folk homes," and other places.

3. Possibly the most extensive collection of letters from Carville
is in the possession of the Landry and Manes families of New Iberia,
Louisiana. These letters were written by two brothers to members
of their family between 1919 and 1932. I will address these letters
and family responses to these letters in the final chapter on
"Postmemory."

4. This date is probably an error. Ramirez says elsewhere that he
entered Carville in 1968, and he was diagnosed shortly before.

5. Caruth says that the centrality and complexity of trauma in the twentieth century was first addressed by Freud in *Beyond the Pleasure Principle* (individual trauma) and in *Moses and Monotheism* (historical trauma). She says these works form the basis for "Freud's formulation of trauma as a theory of the peculiar incomprehensibility of human survival" (1996: 58).

6. This would not be so for those who died at Carville before the 1940s, never having the benefit of effective treatment or cure.

7. As Susan J. Brison points out, "Survivors of trauma frequently remark that they are not the same people they were before they were traumatized" (1999: 39). She adds, "The undoing of the self in trauma involves a radical disruption of memory, a severing of past from present and, typically, an inability to envision a future. And yet trauma survivors often eventually find ways to reconstruct themselves and carry on the reconfigured lives" (39). While there is not the radical disruption of memory for leprosy patients, much of what she says here does apply to former Carville patients.

8. For more on this topic, see "Reviving and Resisting a Termination Model" by Janet Franz (1992), who argues that the federal government succumbed to political and emotional pressure to maintain the HD Center at Carville long after it was politically or financially feasible to do so. Franz has further examined the federal government's role at Carville in a presentation entitled "Policy Making in a Garbage Can" (2000).

Chapter 3. "Through the Hole in the Fence"

1. Writing in 1997, William Ian Miller says in *The Anatomy of Disgust*, after quoting a passage from *Life of St. Anselm* (ca. 1090): "Let us put aside for the moment the revulsion that lepers evoke, which is perfectly understandable to us" (149–50).

2. Louis Boudreaux died in 1986 and is buried in the Carville graveyard.

3. Martin used the term "burnt-out cases" in her 1950 best-seller, *Miracle at Carville*, to describe leprosy patients whose disease was

arrested or in remission only after they were already severely impaired or disabled. Graham Greene uses *A Burnt-Out Case* as the title of his 1961 novel set in a "leproserie" in Africa. Greene's title refers to leprosy patients who have suffered great loss, particularly loss of sensation, but are no longer infectious. In the novel, the African character Deo Gratias has "lost all his toes and fingers" but is no longer an active case (13). Greene's title is also a metaphor for Querry, the main character who comes to Africa as a disillusioned world-famous architect. Greene does not acknowledge Martin's book as the source of his title, and it is unclear whether this term was used, in general, in this context before Martin's book. It should be noted that Greene's critically acclaimed novel was given scathing reviews in *The Star* and in other publications by leprologists. It was called insensitive, sensationalistic, a disregard for truth and good taste, and "a travesty of the disease and modern methods of treatment" (see especially Cochran 1961).

4. Betty Martin writes about the first time she was permitted to leave Carville with a pass for a brief visit to New Orleans in December 1928: "I was one of the first of Carville's patients to be given the privilege. Previously leave was granted a patient only in an emergency, such as a serious illness or death in the family and then the patient had to be accompanied, going and returning, by a hospital guard whose expenses the patient or his family had to pay" (1950: 42).

5. Last name omitted by her request. Rita died at Carville in 1989.

6. Chester Carville (Nippy's husband and James's father) was postmaster at the Carville, Louisiana, post office. Mary's husband, Darryl, was postmaster at the Carville Point Clair Post Office Branch on the hospital "station." Darryl was also the first patient to serve on the board of directors of the Iberville Bank in nearby St. Gabriel, and he was well respected in the surrounding community. In James Carville's keynote address at the 1994 Carville Centennial Celebration, he referred to Darryl as "my daddy's best friend." In an article in *The Star* titled "L. A. Carville from Carville, La.," the Carville family is credited with fostering better understanding in the area about Hansen's

disease in the early twentieth century: "Through the Carvilles' deal-ings with the 'home' and by their reassurances to the members of the community, the resentment and phobia gradually began to break down" (1954: 11). L. A. Carville, James Carville's grandfather, had been postmaster from 1908 to 1945. Chester Carville became post-master in 1945.

Chapter 4. Telling It Slant

1. Billy was also a very good pool player. A 1983 article by Jeanne Landry in the *Beaumont Enterprise*, entitled "Leprosy victim remains 'on cue,'" features Billy as a pool player, and says, "Billy Burton, also known as 'Wild Bill from Jacksonville,' carefully bends over his pool cue." The article includes a photo of Billy with his pool cue and the byline, "Billy Burton meticulously tapes one of his hands to his cue" (Landry 1983: 1A).

2. Goffman uses the term *fabrications* for the first-person tall tales in which "the intentional effort of one or more individuals [is] to manage activity so that a party of one or more others will be induced to have a false belief about what it is that is going on" (1974: 83).

3. See also Bauman 1987: 219 for an account of storyteller Ed Bell doing something similar with his audience.

Chapter 5. The World Downside Up

1. For more on medieval leprosy, see Peter Richards's *The Medieval Leper* (1977) and Saul Nathaniel Brody's *The Disease of the Soul: Leprosy in Medieval Literature* (1974).

2. My ideas about the carnivalesque are based primarily upon the work of Mikhail Bakhtin, as well as Barbara Babcock's 1978 work on symbolic inversion, Victor Turner's work on festival (1982a, 1982b, 1987), and Stallybrass and White on transgression (1986).

3. For more on the New Orleans urban Mardi Gras, see Kinser 1990, Roach 1993, and de Caro and Ireland 1988. The Carville Mardi Gras

does not have anything analogous to the New Orleans Mardi Gras Black Indian tribes.

4. Although Carville's doubloons are based on the New Orleans carnival doubloon tradition, real doubloons are obsolete Spanish gold coins. It is interesting to compare the Carville tradition with the 1957 carnival at Palo Seco Hansen's Disease Hospital, Balboa, Canal Zone (operated at that time by Canal Zone Government and Republic of Panama):

> The patients danced every night during the four days of carnival, until daybreak on Ash Wednesday, a Panamanian custom. At dawn they went up the hill dancing and carrying the musical instruments, lingering in the area before the home of Dr. and Mrs. Hurwitz and while they danced, the Hurwitzes threw coins to them, an old Spanish custom. Dr. and Mrs. Hurwitz joined the patients. Mrs. Hurwitz, wearing her montuna, accompanied them to the mess hall where hot coffee was served. The patients continued to dance until just before the sound of the church bells when they symbolically "buried the fish," terminating the festivities. Then they all attended mass, coming out with a cross of ashes on their foreheads. [Ezra Hurwitz was medical superintendent of the hospital.] (Carnival at Palo Seco 1957: 13)

5. The discovery of naturally occurring leprosy in nine-banded armadillos was, in fact, reported in 1977 (Trautman 1985: 12). The belief that armadillos in the wild can carry leprosy is also known in South America. In Mario Vargas Llosa's novel *The Storyteller*, a character says, "I've always known that armadillo meat must not be eaten because the armadillo has an impure mother and brings harm; spots come out all over the body of anybody who eats it" (1989: 49). Vargas Llosa has acknowledged his allusions to leprosy, although he does not mention it by name.

6. It is interesting to note Turner's comments on masks in another context (referring to masked dancers in the Ndembu circumcision ritual, *Mukanda*): "*Makishi* (maskers) among the Ndembu, etc., demand

food and gifts as a right. Optation pervades the liminoid phenomenon, obligation the liminal. One is all play and choice, and entertainment, the other is a matter of deep seriousness, even dread; it is demanding, compulsory, though, indeed, fear provokes nervous laughter from the women (who, if touched by the *makishi*, are believed to contract leprosy, become sterile, or go mad!)" (1982a: 43).

Chapter 6. "Under the Pecans"

1. An article on Louis Boudreaux's life and death was published in Louisiana State University's student newspaper, the *Daily Reveille*, on November 13, 1986. The article, by T. Bradley Keith, was entitled "Louis Boudreaux: a life of pain, achievement." The article included a photograph of his gravestone with the name "Louis A. Houillon."

Chapter 7. Remembering Leprosy

1. The National Hansen's Disease Museum is open Monday through Friday, from 10:00 A.M. to noon and from 1:00 to 4:00 P.M., for tours. The museum's first curator is Elizabeth Schexnyder. For more information about the museum, visit the website at http://www.bphc.hrsa.gov/nhdp/NHD_MUSEUM_HISTORY.htm.

The museum, funded by the NHDP and by grants from the Louisiana Endowment for the Humanities and other sources, is also listed on the Iberville Parish Tourist Commission website.

2. In *Defacement: Public Secrecy and the Labor of the Negative*, Michael Taussig raises the question, "Yet what if the truth is not so much a secret as a *public* secret, as is the case with most important social knowledge, *knowing what not to know*?" (1999: 2, italics in original). Taussig defines *public secret* as *"that which is generally known, but cannot be articulated."* (5, italics in original). It seems likely that the diagnosis of leprosy and residence at Carville were often public secrets, things that were known but that no one spoke openly about in public.

Sources Cited and Consulted

Abrahams, Roger D. 1987. An American Vocabulary of Celebration. In *Time Out of Time: Essays on the Festival*. Ed. Alessandro Falassi, pp. 173–83. Albuquerque: University of New Mexico Press.

Ariès, Philippe. 1974. *Western Attitudes Toward Death*. Baltimore: Johns Hopkins University Press.

Babcock, Barbara A. 1977. The Story in the Story: Metanarration in Folk Narrative. In *Verbal Art as Performance*. Ed. Richard Bauman, pp. 61–79. Prospect Heights, Ill.: Waveland Press.

Babcock, Barbara A., ed. 1978. *The Reversible World: Symbolic Inversion in Art and Society*. Ithaca and London: Cornell University Press.

Baddeley, Alan. 1990. *Human Memory: Theory and Practice*. Boston and London: Allyn and Bacon.

Bai, Matt. 1999. The Only World They Knew. *Newsweek*, Mar. 29: 68–69.

Bakhtin, Mikhail. 1984 [1968]. *Rabelais and His World*. Trans. Helene Iswolksy. Bloomington: Indiana University Press.

Bateson, Mary Catherine. 1990. *Composing a Life*. New York: Plume.

Bauman, Richard. 1972. The La Have Island General Store: Sociability and Verbal Art in a Nova Scotia Community. *Journal of American Folklore* 85: 330–41.

———. 1986. *Story, Performance, and Event: Contextual Studies of Oral Narratives*. Cambridge: Cambridge University Press.

————. 1987. Ed Bell, Texas Storyteller: The Framing and Reframing of Life Experience. *Journal of Folklore Research* 24 (3): 197–221.

Ben-Amos, Dan. 1976. Talmudic Tall Tales. In *Folklore Today: A Festschrift for Richard M. Dorson*. Ed. Linda Degh, Henry Glassie, and Felix J. Oinas. Bloomington: Indiana University Press.

Bermudez, Rafael. 1976. Hansen's Disease Facility Offers Up-to-Date Service. *Enid* [Okla.] *Morning News*, Apr. 11: B-8.

Billy. 1986. Personal interview. Carville, La. Mar. 27.

Boudreaux, Louis. 1983. Personal interview. Carville, La. Dec.

Bragg, Rick. 1995. The Last Lepers. *New York Times*, June 19: pp. A1 and A7.

Brison, Susan J. 1999. Trauma, Narratives and the Remaking of the Self. In *Acts of Memory: Cultural Recall in the Present*. Ed. Mieke Bal, Jonathan Crewe, and Leo Spitzer, pp. 39–54. Hanover and London: Dartmouth College (University Press of New England).

Brody, Saul Nathaniel. 1974. *The Disease of the Soul: Leprosy in Medieval Literature*. Ithaca and London: Cornell University Press.

Brown, R., and J. Kulik. 1977. Flashbulb Memories. *Cognition* 5: 73–99.

Broyard, Anatole. 1992. *Intoxicated by My Illness and Other Writings on Life and Death*. Ed. Alexandra Broyard. New York: Clarkson Potter.

Burgess, Perry. 1940. *Who Walks Alone*. New York: Henry Holt.

Calandro, Charles H. 1983. From Disgrace to Dignity—The Louisiana Leprosy Home, 1894–1921. Unpublished master's thesis, Louisiana State University.

Carnival at Palo Seco. 1957. *The Star* 16 (4): 13.

Caruth, Cathy, ed. 1995. *Trauma: Explorations in Memory*. Baltimore: Johns Hopkins University Press.

Caruth, Cathy. 1996. *Unclaimed Experiences: Trauma, Narration and History*. Baltimore: Johns Hopkins University Press.

Clements, William M. 1980. Personal Narrative, the Interview Context, and the Question of Tradition. *Western Folklore* 34: 106–12.

Clinton, Ed. 1957. Mardi Gras at Carville Sparkles with Gaiety. *Baton Rouge State Times*, Mar. 6: p. 1.

Cochrane, Robert C., M.D. 1961. Dr. Cochrane Reviews Graham Greene's New Book for *The Star*. *The Star* 20 (4): 10–11.

Conway, Martin A. 1990. *Autobiographical Memory: An Introduction*. Philadelphia: Open University Press.

Crocker, J. C. 1982. Ceremonial Masks. In *Celebration: Studies in Festivity and Ritual*. Ed. Victor Turner, pp. 77–88. Washington, D.C.: Smithsonian Institution Press

Crouch, Howard E., and Sister Mary Augustine. 1989. *Two Hearts, One Fire: A Glimpse Behind the Mask of Leprosy*. New York: Damien-Dutton Society.

Culbertson, Roberta. 1995. Embodied Memory, Transcendence, and Telling: Recounting Trauma, Re-establishing the Self. *New Literary History* 26: 169–95.

de Caro, F. A., and Tom Ireland. 1988. Every Man a King: Worldview, Social Tension and Carnival in New Orleans. *International Folklore Review* 6: 58–66.

Degh, Linda, and Andrew Vazsonyi. 1974. The Memorate and the Proto-Memorate. *Journal of American Folklore* 87: 225–49.

Douglas, Mary. 1991. Witchcraft and Leprosy: Two Strategies of Exclusion. *Man* 26 (4): 723–46.

Drakos, Georg. 1992. The Woman Who Wouldn't Abandon Her Leprous Husband. *Tradisjon* 22: 27–43.

———. 1997a. History, Intertextuality, and Social Power: Leprosy and Self-Understanding in Late Twentieth Century Greece. American Folklore Society Meeting Presentation, Austin, Texas.

———. 1997b. *Makt över kropp och hälsa: om leprasjukas självförståelse i dagens Grekland. [Empowering body and health: Leprosy and self-understanding in late twentieth century Greece.]* Stockholm/Stehag. Östling bokförlag Symposion. (Diss.)

Ell, Stephen R. 1986. Leprosy and Social Class in the Middle Ages. *International Journal of Leprosy* 54 (2): 300–305.

Elwood, Julia Rivera, ed. 1994. *Known simply to the rest of the world as Carville . . . 100 years*. Carville, La.: Department of Health and

Human Services, U.S. Public Health Service, Gillis W. Long National Hansen's Disease Center.

———. 1996. *With Love in Their Hearts: The Sisters of St. Vincent de Paul 1896–1996.* Carville, La.: Department of Health and Human Services, U.S. Public Health Service, Gillis W. Long National Hansen's Disease Center.

Elwood, Julia. 1975. "One Disastrous Phrase." *The Star.* 34 (3): 6.

———. 1983–99. Personal interviews. Carville, La. Dec. 1983; Feb. 1984; July 31, 1989; July 13, 1995; July 17, 1997; Apr. 13, June 26, and Oct. 22, 1998; May 1999.

Elwood, Ray. 1975. Man in Demand. *The Star* 35 (1): 8–10.

———. 1984, 1986. Personal interviews. Carville, La.

Enna, Carl D., M.D., and Charles F. Byrd. 1975. "The History and Development of the National Leprosarium in the United States." Taken from *International Surgery*, Section 2, Oct. 1969; reprinted in *The Star* 90 (6) [Nov./Dec. 1975].

Epstein, Julia. 1995. *Altered Conditions: Disease, Medicine, and Storytelling.* New York: Routledge.

Falassi, Alessandro, ed. 1987. *Time Out of Time: Essays on the Festival.* Albuquerque: University of New Mexico Press.

Foucault, Michel. 1988 (1961). *Madness and Civilization: A History of Insanity in the Age of Reason.* Trans. Richard Howard. New York: Vintage Books.

Frantz, Janet. 1992. Reviving and Resisting a Termination Model. *Policy Sciences* 25: 175–89.

———. 2000. The National Leprosarium: Policy Making in a Garbage Can. Unpublished presentation. University of Louisiana at Lafayette.

———. 2002. Political Resources for Policy Terminators. *Policy Studies Journal* 30: 11–38.

From Carville With Hope. 1965. [Booklet published by *The Star* staff, p. 11.]

Gaudet, Marcia. 1984. Folklore and Compassion: The Treatment of Leprosy in George Washington Cable's "Jean-Ah Poquelin." *Louisiana Literature* 1 (2): 20–22.

———. 1988. Through the Hole in the Fence: Personal Narratives of Absconding from Carville. *Fabula* 29: 354–64.

———. 1990. Telling It Slant: Personal Narratives, Tall Tales, and the Reality of Leprosy. *Western Folklore* 49: 191–207.

———. 1998. The World Downside Up: Mardi Gras at Carville. *Journal of American Folklore* 111: 23–38.

Gilman, Sander. 1988. *Disease and Representation.* Ithaca: Cornell University Press.

———. 1995. *Picturing Health and Illness: Images of Identity and Difference.* Baltimore: Johns Hopkins University Press.

Goffman, Erving. 1963. *Stigma: Notes on the Management of Spoiled Identity.* Englewood Cliffs, N.J.: Prentice-Hall.

———. 1979. *Frame Analysis.* New York: Harper & Row.

Gosnell, Lynn, and Suzanne Gott. 1989. San Fernando Cemetery: Decorations of Love and Loss in a Mexican-American Community. In *Cemeteries and Grave Markers: Voices of American Culture.* Ed. Richard E. Meyer, pp. 217–36. Ann Arbor: UMI Research Press.

Gould, Cynthia M. 1991. Sister Hilary Ross and Carville: Her Thirty-Seven Year Struggle Against Hansen's Disease. M.A. thesis, University of New Orleans.

Grön, K. 1973. Leprosy in Literature and Art. *International Journal of Leprosy* 41 (2): 249–83.

Gussow, Zachary. 1979. Notes on the History of Leprosy in Louisiana. *Southern Medical Journal* 72 (5): 600–604.

———. 1989. *Leprosy, Racism and Public Health: Social Policy in Chronic Disease.* Boulder: Westview Press.

Gussow, Zachary, and George S. Tracy. 1968. Status, Ideology, and Adaptation to Stigmatized Illness: A Study of Leprosy. *Human Organization* 27: 316–25.

———. 1971. The Use of Archival Materials in the Analysis and Interpretation of Field Data: A Case Study in the Institutionalization of the Myth of Leprosy as "Leper." *American Anthropologist* 73 (3): 695–709.

Hannah, Barry. 1995. Old Terror, New Hearts. *The Oxford American*. Oct./Nov.: 40–49.

Harding Susan. 1991. Representing Fundamentalism: The Problem of the Repugnant Cultural Other. *Social Research* 58: 373–93.

Harmon, Johnny. 1996. *King of the Microbes: The Autobiography of Johnny P. Harmon*. Baton Rouge: n.p.

Hayakawa, S. I. 1972. *Language in Thought and Action*, 3rd ed. New York: Harcourt, Brace, Jovanovich.

Hazel. 1984. Personal interview. Carville, La. Jan.

Hirsch, Marianne. 1997. *Family Frames: Photography, Narrative and Postmemory*. Cambridge: Harvard University Press.

———. 1999. Projected Memory: Holocaust Photographs in Personal and Public Fantasy. In *Acts of Memory: Cultural Recall in the Present*. Ed. Mieke Bal, Jonathan Crewe, and Leo Spitzer, pp. 3–23. Hanover: University Press of New England.

Ives, Edward D. 1988. *George Magoon and the Down East Game War*. Urbana: University of Illinois Press.

Jackson, Bruce. 1965. Prison Folklore. *Journal of American Folklore* 78: 317–29.

———. 1972. *In the Life: Versions of the Criminal Experience*. New York: Holt, Rinehart and Winston.

———. 1978. Deviance as Success: The Double Inversion of Stigmatized Roles. In *The Reversible World: Symbolic Inversion in Art and Society*. Ed. Barbara Babcock, pp. 258–75. Ithaca and London: Cornell University Press.

Jacobson, Robert R., M.D. Ph.D. 1990. The Face of Hansen's Disease in the United States. *Arch Dermatol* 126: 1627–30.

Johnson, Sarah Spell. 2001. Family's Letters Shape Poetry. *Advocate*, July 30: pp. 1B–2B.

Kalisch, Philip A. 1972. The Strange Case of John Early: A Study of the Stigma of Leprosy. *International Journal of Leprosy* 40 (3): 291–305.

———. 1973. Lepers, Anachronisms, and the Progressives: A Study in Stigma, 1889–1920. *Louisiana Studies* 7 (3): 489–531.

Kendall, John Smith. 1954. "What Led to Founding the Carville Hospital: A Little Known Chapter." *The Star* 14 (3): 17–18.

Kinser, Samuel. 1990. *Carnival, American Style: Mardi Gras at New Orleans and Mobile.* Chicago and London: University of Chicago Press.

Kirshenblatt-Gimblett, Barbara. 1989a. Authoring Lives. *Journal of Folklore Research* 26: 123 50.

———. 1989b. Objects of Memory: Material Culture as Life Review. In *Folk Groups and Folklore Genres: A Reader.* Ed. Elliott Oring, pp. 278–85. Logan: Utah State University Press.

Klymasz, Robert B. 1983. Folklore of the Canadian-Border. In *Handbook of American Folklore.* Ed. Richard M. Dorson, pp. 227–32. Bloomington: Indiana University Press.

Kniffen, Fred. 1967. Necrogeography in the United States. *Geographical Review* 57: 426–27.

L. A. Carville from Carville, La. 1954. *The Star* 14 (3): 11.

Labov, William, and Joshua Waletzky. 1967. Narrative Analysis: Oral Versions of Personal Experience. In *Essays on the Verbal and Visual Arts.* Ed. June Helm, pp. 12–44. Seattle: University of Washington Press.

Landry, Jeanne. 1983. Leprosy victim remains "on cue." *Beaumont Enterprise*, Sept. 6: pp. 1A and 6A.

Langellier, Kristin M. 1989. Personal Narratives: Perspectives on Theory and Research. *Text and Performance Quarterly* 9 (4): 243–76.

Lewis, Gilbert. 1987. A Lesson From Leviticus: Leprosy. *Man* 22: 593–612.

Macgregor, F., et al. 1953. *Facial Deformities and Plastic Surgery.* Springfield, Ill.: Charles C. Thomas.

Man in Demand. 1975 *The Star* 35 (1): 8–10.

Manes, Christopher Lee. 2001. *Regardez.* Lafayette: Creative Writing Chapbook, University of Louisiana at Lafayette, Department of English.

———. 2003a. In the Name of Whom It Was Said, *Regardez*. M.A. thesis, University of Louisiana at Lafayette.

———. 2003b. Regarding Carville: The Letters of Norbert and Edmond Landry. *Louisiana History* 44 (3): 325–38.

Manes, Claire. 2003. In His Own Hand—The Correspondence of Edmond G. Landry from Carville, Louisiana. Unpublished presentation. Louisiana Folklore Society Meeting, Lafayette, Apr. 5.

Manes, Leonide Landry. 2000. Personal interview, New Iberia, La. Aug. 18.

Mardi Gras at Carville Sparkles with Gaity. 1957. *The Star* 16 (4): 8–9.

Martin, Betty. 1950. *Miracle at Carville*. Ed. Evelyn Wells. New York: Image Books.

———. 1959. *No One Must Ever Know*. Ed. Evelyn Wells. New York: Doubleday.

Martin, Betty, and Harry Martin. 1995. Personal interview. Carville, La., July 13.

Mary Ruth. 2001. Personal interview. Carville, La. Apr. 6.

———. 2002. Personal interview. Carville, La. July 26.

Meyers, Richard. 1993. "Strangers in a Strange Land": Ethnic Cemeteries in America. In *Ethnicity and the American Cemetery*. Ed. Richard E. Meyers, pp. 1–13. Bowling Green, Ohio: BGSU Popular Press.

McKinney, Joan. 1997. Administration bill paves way for Carville job-training center. *Advocate*, June 12: p. 22-A.

Mesnil, Marianne. 1976. The Masked Festival: Disguise or Affirmation? *Culture* (Festivals and Culture Issue) 3 (2): 11–29.

Miller, William Ian. 1997. *The Anatomy of Disgust*. Cambridge: Harvard University Press.

Mizell-Nelson, Michael. 2003. Treated as Lepers: The Patient-Led Reform Movement at the National Leprosarium, 1931–46. *Louisiana History* 44 (3): 301–24.

Morris, David B. 1998. *Illness and Culture in the Postmodern Age*. Berkeley and Los Angeles: University of California Press.

Morrison, Toni. 1984. Memory, Creation, and Writing. *Thought* 59: 385–90.

Myerhoff, Barbara. 1979. *Number Our Days*. New York: E. P. Dutton.

Nakagawa, Tadashi. 1987. The Cemetery as Cultural Manifestation: Louisiana Necrogeopraphy. Ph.D. diss. Louisiana State University.

Napier, A. David. 1986. *Masks, Transformations and Paradox*. Berkeley and Los Angeles: University of California Press.

———. 1987. Festival Masks: A Typology. In *Time Out of Time*. Ed. Alessandro Falassi, pp. 211–19.

National Leprosarium. 1948. *The Star* 8 (4): 2–16.

Navon, Liora. 1995. From Wordless Ritual to Ritual Words: An Analysis of Ritualized Contact with Leprosy. *Anthropos* 90: 511–24.

Neisser, Ulric, ed. 1982. *Memory Observed: Remembering in Natural Contexts*. San Francisco: W. H. Freeman.

Nelson, Hilde Lindeman. 2001. *Damaged Identities: Narrative Repair*. Ithaca: Cornell University Press.

Nicolaisen, W. F. H. 1993. Why Tell Stories About Innocent, Persecuted Heroines? *Western Folklore* 52: 61–71.

Oring, Elliott. 1987. Generating Lives: The Contruction of an Autobiography. *Journal of Folklore Research* 24: 241–62.

Page, Ann. 1944. The Ladies. *The Star* 14 (3): 28–29, 31.

Paz, C. J. 1990. The Use of Philippine Folklore in WHO Scientific Research. Unpublished paper. University of the Philippines.

Pope, John. 2002. Johnny Harmon, 90, Lived with Leprosy. *Times-Picayune*, Sept. 28: p. B5.

Ramadanovic, Petar. 2000. *Forgetting Futures: On Memory, Trauma, and Identity*. Lanham, Md.: Lexington Books.

Ramircz, Jose, Jr. 2002. Leprosy—The L-Word. The Nippon Foundation. <http://www.nippon-foundation.or.jp/eng/current/>

———. Forthcoming. *Squint*. N.p.

Reeves, Sally K., and William D. 1993–94. Carville: A Century's Worth of Miracles. *Louisiana Life* (Winter): 46–51.

Richards, Peter. 1977. *The Medieval Leper: And His Northern Heirs*. Cambridge, England: D. S. Brewer; Totowa, N.J.: Rowman and Littlefield.

Risse, Guenter B., M.D., Ph.D. 1999. *Mending Bodies, Saving Souls: A History of Hospitals*. New York: Oxford University Press.

Rita. 1983, 1984. Personal interviews. Carville, La. Dec. 1983, Jan. 1984.

Roach, Joseph. 1993. Carnival and the Law in New Orleans. *Drama Review* 37 (3): 42–75.

Roberts, Penny Brown. 1998. At the End of the Road: Closing Louisiana's Leprosy Home. *Lafayette Advertiser*, July 27, 1998: pp. 1B and 3B.

Robinson, John. 1981. Personal Narratives Reconsidered. *Journal of American Folklore* 94: 58–85.

Robinson, Ray. 1984. The Leper and the Bear Hunter. *Cajun Tales of the Louisiana Bayous*, pp. 45–48. Gray, La.: Cypress Publishers.

Rogers, Patrick, and Kate Klise. 1999. Cast Away: Betty Martin's Fearful Illness Meant a Sentence to Exile. *People*, May 24: 163–66.

Ross, Sister Hilary. 1936. Unpublished journal. National Hansen's Disease Center Archives. Carville, La.

Rutledge. C. M. 1970. Treatment Models and Patient Adaptation: A Study of Life in a Leprosarium. M.A. thesis. Louisiana State University, Baton Rouge.

Sabin, Thomas D. 1981. The Penikese Hospital. *The Star* 41 (1): 10–11. (Reprinted from *New England Journal of Medicine* 304: 1610–12.)

Salaman, Ester. 1982. A Collection of Moments. In *Memory Observed*. Ed. Ulric Neisser, pp. 49–65. San Francisco: W. H. Freeman.

Salvaggio, John, M.D. 1992. *New Orleans Charity Hospital: A Story of Physicians, Politics, and Poverty*. Baton Rouge: Louisiana State University Press.

Santino, Jack. 1995. *All Around the Year: Holidays and Celebrations in American Life*. Urbana and Chicago: University of Illinois Press.

Sapir, J. David. 1981. Leper, Hyena, and Blacksmith in Kujamaat Diola Thought. *American Ethnologist* 813: 526–43.

Saxon, Lyle. 1988 [1929]. *Fabulous New Orleans*. New Orleans: Pelican Publishing.

Schatzlein, Joanne, and Daniel P. Sulmasy. 1988. Diagnosis of St. Francis: Evidence for Leprosy. *Franciscan Studies* 47: 181–217.

Silla, Eric. 1998. *People Are Not the Same: Leprosy and Identity in Twentieth-Century Mali*. Portsmouth, N.H.: Heinemann.

Silvers, Jonathan. 1999. Last Days at the Leprosarium. *Life Magazine*, Apr.: 96–100.

Singer, Milton. 1972. *When a Great Tradition Modernizes: An Anthropological Approach to Indian Civilization*. New York: Praeger Publisher.

Skinsnes, Olaf K., and Robert M. Elvove. 1970. Leprosy in Society V. "Leprosy" in Occidental Literature. *International Journal of Leprosy* 38 (3): 294–307.

Sloane, David Charles. 1991. *The Last Great Necessity: Cemeteries in American History*. Baltimore: Johns Hopkins University Press.

Smith, Robert J. 1972. Festivals and Celebrations. In *Folklore and Folklife*. Ed. Richard M. Dorson, pp. 159–72. Chicago: University of Chicago Press.

Smith, Thomas Hunter. 2003. Do Unto Others: Persecution and Miracle at Louisiana's Leprosy Hospital, 1894–2003. Paper presented at Louisiana Historical Association Meeting, Mar. 28, Lafayette.

Snyder, Sharon L., Brenda Jo Brueggemann, and Rosemarie Garland-Thomson. 2002. *Disability Studies: Enabling the Humanities*. New York: Modern Language Association of American.

Sontag, Susan. 1978. *Illness as Metaphor*. New York: Farrar, Straus and Giroux.

———. 1989. *AIDS and Its Metaphors*. New York: Farrar, Straus and Giroux.

Stahl, Sandra K. Dolby. 1977. The Personal Narrative as Folklore. *Journal of the Folklore Institute* 14: 9–30.

———. 1983. Personal Experience Stories. In *Handbook of American Folklore*. Ed. Richard Dorson, pp. 268–76. Bloomington: Indiana University Press.

Stallybrass, Peter, and Allon White. 1986. *The Politics and Poetics of Transgression*. London: Methuen.

Stanley, Laurie C. C. 1982. *Unclean! Unclean!: Leprosy in New Brunswick, 1844–80*. Moncton, N.B.: Les Editions d'Acadie.

Stanley-Blackwell, Laurie. 1988. Leprosy in New Brunswick, 1844–1910: A Reconsideration. Ph.D. diss. Queen's University.

Stanley-Blackwell, Laurie C. C. 1993. The Mysterious Stranger and the Acadian Good Samaritan: Leprosy Folklore in Nineteenth-Century New Brunswick. *Acadiensis* 22 (2): 27–39.

Stein, Stanley. 1963. *Alone No Longer*. New York: Funk and Wagnalls.

Stoeltje, Beverly J., and Richard Bauman. 1988. The Semiotics of Folklore Performance. In *The Semiotic Web 1987*. Ed. Thomas E. Sebeok and Jean Umiker-Sebeok, pp. 585–99. Berlin: Mouton de Gruyter.

Stricker, Sister Laura. 1984. Personal interview. Carville, La. Jan.

Tallant, Robert. 1976 [1947]. *Mardi Gras*. Gretna, La.: Pelican Publishing.

Taussig, Michael T. 1999. *Defacement: Public Secrecy and the Labor of the Negative*. Stanford: Stanford University Press.

Theroux, Paul. 1994. The Lepers of Moyo. *Granta* 48: 127–91.

Thomassie, Tanya. 2004. Personal e-mail communication. Jan. 8.

Trautman, John R., M.D. 1985. A Brief History of Hansen's Disease. *The Star* 45 (2): 10–12.

———. 1989. Epidemiological Aspects of Hansen's Disease (HD). *The Star* 49 (2). (Reprinted in pamphlet form.)

———. n.d. *Some Questions Commonly Asked About Hansen's Disease . . . and Some Concise Answers*. Carville, La.: National Hansen's Disease Center.

Turner, Victor. 1982a. *From Ritual to Theatre: The Human Seriousness of Play*. New York: Performing Arts Journal Publications.

———, ed. 1982b. *Celebration: Studies in Festivity and Ritual*. Washington, D.C.: Smithsonian Institution Press.

———. 1987. Carnival, Ritual and Play in Rio de Janeiro. In *Time Out of Time: Essays on the Festival*. Ed. Alessandro Falassi. pp. 74–90. Albuquerque: University of New Mexico Press.

Vargas Llosa, Mario. 1989. *The Storyteller*. Translated by Helen Lane. New York: Penguin Books.

White, Cassandra. 2001. Cultural Aspects of Leprosy Treatment in Rio de Janeiro, Brazil. Ph.D. diss. Tulane University.

———. 2002. Sociocultural Considerations in the Treatment of Leprosy in Rio de Janeiro, Brazil. *Leprosy Review* 73 (4): 356–65.

———. 2003. Carville and Curupaiti: Experiences of Confinement and Community. *História, Ciências, Saúde-Manguinhos* 10 (1): 123–41.

Documentary Films/Television Presentations

Banished: Living with Leprosy. 1999. Produced for the Discovery Channel by Phyllis Ward & Associates. 50 minutes.

Exiles in Their Own Country: The Long Road Back. 1994. G. W. Long Hansen's Disease Center. 60 minutes.

Secret People. 1998. John Anderson and Laura Harrison, co-producers. 60 minutes.

Unlikely Heroes. In production. Sally Squires and John Wilhelm.

Works of Literature

Atwood, Margaret. 1994. Dance of the Lepers. In *Good Bones and Small Murders*. New York: Doubleday/Nan A. Talese.

Blackburn, Julia. 1999. *The Leper's Companions*. New York: Pantheon Books.

Greene, Graham. 1961. *A Burnt-Out Case*. New York: Viking.

London, Jack. 1912a. Koloau the Leper. In *The House of Pride and Other Tales of Hawaii*. New York: Macmillan.

———. 1912b. The Sheriff of Kona. In *The House of Pride and Other Tales of Hawaii*. New York: Macmillan.

Maalouf, Amin. 1988. *Leo Africanus*. Trans. Peter Sluglett. New York: New Amsterdam Books.

Merwin, W. S. 1998. *The Folding Cliffs: A Narrative of 19th-century Hawaii*. New York: Alfred A. Knopf.

Newth, Mette. 1998. *The Dark Light*. Trans. Faith Ingwersen. New York: Farrar Straus & Giraud.

Tsukiyama, Gail. 1995. *The Samurai's Garden*. New York: St. Martin's Press.

Updike, John. 1978. From the Journal of a Leper. *New Yorker*. July 17. pp. 28–33.

Vargas-Llosa. Mario. 1968. *The Green House*. Trans. Gregory Rabassa. New York: Farrar, Straus and Giroux.

———. 1989. *The Storyteller*. Trans. Helen Lane. New York: Penguin Books.

Index